GOD KNOWS
I WON'T BE FAT
AGAIN

GOD KNOWS
I WON'T BE FAT
AGAIN

KAREN WISE

Thomas Nelson Publishers
Nashville • New York

Third printing

Copyright 1978 by Karen Wise

Library of Congress Cataloging in Publication Data

Wise, Karen.
  God knows I won't be fat again.

  Includes index.
  1. Obesity. 2. Reducing. 3. Christian life—1960-
I. Title.
RC628.W53   613.2'5   78-10517
ISBN 0-8407-5665-8

I dedicate this book to those people who, without ever losing sight of my potential, touched my life at strategic times, displaying a love and concern for me . . . just as I was:

Dertha T. Shooks
Linda Love
George and Margrett Poole
John W. Peterson
Louise Chamberlain
John Haggai

CONTENTS

FOREWORD

When word got out that I would soon be a father, many hinted that such a fact would change my life. It did. It has. It continues to do so.

I have written several things for Karen: excuse slips to be read by teachers, funny little speeches for her to read at banquets, and a few checks for life's inevitable expenses. But a foreword for a book about her own life, struggles, and triumphs is a task for which I am not fully prepared or equipped.

I am sure Karen has learned something about herself in the stark reality of words staring back at her from these pages. You can never escape the words you write through prayer and tears. They are part of you. This story, as is Karen herself, is also part of me, my life, my ministry, my marriage, my faith.

Some chapters are difficult for Karen's mother and me to read. We are participants, not just spectators. Other parents will find themselves sketched in this record. We hope it shall not be construed that our dedication to God and His service was too great, too complete. Between the lines it should be read that dedication is not a substitute for wisdom; that consecration to self and ambition may be confused with consecration to the Lord.

It takes a little getting used to—to read about a daughter you have known and loved all her life, to read a story you know very well and yet to discover that you do not know it all. At times, it is a stranger's tale, a lightning bolt on a dark landscape. Then again, you want to rewrite it as you saw it. There are long paragraphs, very important ones to me, that Karen doesn't seem to know were there.

No life can be set forth in each detail on pages of a book. Karen's life didn't develop with the clarity of words punctuated with small marks. It happened in love and tears, in hopes and fears, in silence and thunder. It happened in talent and fact, in vision and despair, in pride and anger. Now that these chapters are written, I sense some of John's joy: "I have no greater joy than to hear that my children walk in truth" (3 John 4).

Everyone who knows Karen utters a prayer of gratitude for her unbelievable victory over excess weight. There is a phrase that seems appropriate. I have said it several times.

"Who will care for this child?"

Answer: "Her mother and I."

"Who will pay for the music lessons?"

Answer: "Her mother and I."

"Who will sign for her driver's license?"

Answer: "Her mother and I."

"Who prays for Karen?"

Answer: "Her mother and I."
"Who gives Karen to be married to Larry?"
Answer: "Her mother and I."
"Who rejoices that Karen is thin?"
Answer: "Her mother and I."

Dr. Louis Paul Lehman

CHAPTER 1

I LIKE IT! I LIKE IT!

Driving north on I-85 in Atlanta a few months ago, I pulled into the left lane to pass a truck. When I was even with the cab, the driver leaned out his window and whistled at me.

Flushed with excitement and on impulse, I actually leaned across the front seat to see if I could get a good look at him! I guess I wanted to make sure it was really I who had captured his attention.

Suddenly I realized I was not only losing my composure but also drifting off onto the median and losing control of my car. Immediately I sat up straight, got the car back on the freeway, stepped on the gas, and pulled back into the right lane in front of the truck. Still flushed and now very embarrassed, I just laughed out loud as I drove on.

At thirty-five years of age, I had been whistled at for the first time in my life, and I obviously couldn't handle it very well. That man in the truck had no idea how he had made my day. He had no way of knowing what an adjustment it has been to go from 340 pounds to a wolf whistle—at last!

Through four years of dieting, I have said to myself every day, "Karen, you're going to make it this time." And that truck driver, whoever he was (bless him!), evidently agreed that I had.

This is not like other weight books. There are no low-cal recipes or exercise charts included. On these pages are simply the facts of how God, very slowly but effectively, has taken hold of a life cluttered with mistrust, cynicism, hurt, and lots of extra pounds . . . and created a miracle.

I actually have two stories to tell, but both are deeply entwined. One is the story of my eating habit, which eventually controlled every facet of my life and ruined my self-worth, leaving me with only the ability to fail. The other is the story of a preacher's kid growing up in a Christian society, which at times had no room for someone with my personality, my ambitions, and my desires.

I want to share my years of conflict and turmoil—all those years of thinking God had made His *one big mistake* in the way He put me together.

In order to understand me, I will tell you about my parents, my childhood, my Christian world, my marriage, my children, and for a little spice— even my present dress size.

We all need to know that God still works in the lives of *human*, human beings. He doesn't always perform overnight miracles on those of us who fight Him and insist on learning the hard way. If your progress in becoming the person you know God wants you to be seems slow and very difficult, you are not alone.

I have written this book first of all for me. What an experience it has been to write my life down on paper—probably the most helpful and most difficult thing I have ever done. It was not fun plowing through the middle chapters, being reminded of all the wrong choices and dumb mistakes I have made. But it proved to me all over again the goodness of God and the love and patience He has shown toward me. And it has made me appreciate more than ever before the ability that only God has of sweeping up the mistakes, the pain, and the guilt, and throwing them away—and I don't mean just in the wastebasket beside my desk.

I have also written these pages for you, whatever your problem might be. If you have a weight problem of any dimension, I pray that this book will help you. You may not have *that* particular problem, but there are many Christian people who have something in their lives that hinders them from being what God wants them to be—that something you think even God can't handle. It may be a bad habit, a bad temper, an attitude, or an overdose of guilt. It could be anything. I simply want to emphasize in these chapters that God deals in impossibilities.

Or you may be a preacher's kid, an evangelist's kid, or a missionary's kid who is fighting hard to understand a lot of things. You may find yourself hidden in the lines of this book.

And parents, you may be working hard to raise a kid who is like I was, and you may be saying, "What did we do wrong?" You may be throwing up your hands and wondering what you can do to help. You may be rearing children in the Christian world. You may have a talented, noisy, creative child whom you don't know how to handle. You may have an overweight child, and everything you have tried doesn't help. Well, join the group. I have one of both: one that's the actress type and one with a potential weight problem. I think we both can learn something from my past experiences.

What you are about to read is as real as I know how to make it. I couldn't have written it even a year ago without a lot of bitterness, anger, and revenge thrown in. My deepest prayer has been that the book would be free from those things. Just the fact that I can pray that way is a definite sign that God has been hard at work within me.

I still don't have every one of my ducks in a row. I still struggle with some conflicts and periodic low self-esteem. But I've lost 210 pounds, and I am discovering that I am not a slave to Christianity anymore, but a child of God. What a difference!

What God has enabled me to become in comparison to what I was a few years ago is simply marvelous. The future is bright and filled with what God has in store. I want to live every bit of it. And maybe now I can begin to be entrusted with His very best. What a privilege that would be.

"Dear Jesus, I never want to be fat again. Please help me."

CHAPTER 2

LITTLE DID ANYONE KNOW

My father, Dr. Louis Paul Lehman, Jr., was a boy preacher. His career began at the age of nine in Chicago, Illinois, where he, along with his father, Louis Paul Lehman, Sr., and his mother, Florence, attended the well-known Moody Church.

When he was twelve, his only sister Dorothy was born; and shortly afterward my grandfather sold his corner grocery store, and the whole family began traveling in evangelistic meetings from Ohio to Florida.

At thirteen, "Junior Lehman, the boy preacher," as he was called, was licensed to perform marriages, was packing out tabernacles and churches, and was developing quite a reputation as a pulpiteer. In my opinion, he is still one of the greatest preachers in the world. There was no doubt in his mind, even at that early age, that God had called him to preach. He had a great ministry, and many people came to Christ in those meetings.

It is obvious, however, that his life-style was quite different from the normal thirteen-year-old boy's. His father directed the ministry and the

17

music. His mother, a gifted writer and speaker, helped with the writing of the messages and groomed my father's platform ability. My dad preached almost every night and several times on Sunday.

There was little time for riding a bike, climbing a tree, or just hanging around with kids his own age. He simply functioned in another world. He didn't resent being different, for he loved what he was doing. His world demanded daily discipline, study, memorization, and a type of conduct not usually expected of a young boy. He was also privately tutored for a specified number of hours each day.

He lived in an adult world, spent his social hours with adults, and moved from one place to another every few days. Under those circumstances, close friends were rare, and my father was protected a little too much.

As he grew, the organization also grew. The ministry branched out to include a daily radio program, which fast became its main thrust. It was known as the "Bit of Heaven Ministry." People were added to the office staff to answer mail and handle the bookings of meetings. The music staff also grew with the addition of both vocalists and instrumentalists.

The "Bit of Heaven Ministry," heard over WPIT in Pittsburgh and WWVA in Wheeling, West Virginia, both powerful stations, became one of the most popular gospel programs of its day.

My mother, Edna Davis, quit school at age fourteen and left the little coal mining town of

Bridgeville, Pennsylvania, to travel with her brother Harold, who was also a traveling evangelist. My mother played piano and sang with Harold. When Harold married, his wife also became part of the musical team.

Eventually my father's and mother's teams met, and a number of years later my mother was asked to become the pianist for the Lehman evangelistic team. She accepted, in time fell in love with the now grown-up boy preacher, and they were married.

At this time the Lehman team was based in Washington, Pennsylvania. They were on the radio, live, sixteen hours a week, and were holding several one-night meetings a week. The schedule would have broken most people. Up at five o'clock., they started the day with a six o'clock broadcast, followed by rehearsals, more broadcasts, traveling to the night meetings, returning home at midnight or after, and getting up again before daybreak.

My grandparents owned a big three-story house where they provided housing for the staff and traveling evangelists. My great grandmother did most of the cooking, and everyone, including the staff, ate together most of the time. The winters were severe, and no major highways had been built in the hills of Pennsylvania and Ohio. My parents still sit and talk about the nights when they would lie in the snow putting chains on tires or spend hours getting out of a ditch. But they always made it home just in time to do the early morning broadcast.

There were never any vacations, never any days off. Everybody worked seven days a week. You didn't complain, and if you got sick, you worked anyway—like my mother learned to do for nine months. She sat on the piano bench morning after morning, eating soda crackers so she wouldn't get sick during the broadcast. And this is where I entered the picture.

Barely disturbing the flow of all the radio programs, one-night meetings, Sunday afternoon rallies and rehearsals, suddenly a baby girl was born—five pounds, six ounces—just a little thing. They named me Karen Mae. What a bundle of joy I was—or so everybody thought. If they had only known. Or maybe it's just as well we don't know those things ahead of time. One thing is for sure, I was born into a *Christian* world.

Shortly after I was born, a warm and wonderful lady by the name of Pearl Riemer came to live with us. This enabled both of my parents to continue their heavy schedule. We had moved into a red brick house in Washington, Pennsylvania, away from the rest of the family—geographically, anyway. Pearl kept the house shining and kept all my little organdy dresses ironed and ready for my trips from the house. She also loved me deeply, and I guess I never noticed that my folks were gone a lot.

When I was two-and-a-half, I started as part of the team. Dressed in those beautiful organdy dresses, I would stand on a chair behind the pulpit and lead the congregational singing or do a solo number. My Shirley Temple curls and big brown eyes were a winner every time. Even at this age I was aggressive, curious, and well equipped with a strong will and a bad temper—but no extra pounds. I was dainty and cute.

I wasn't afraid of anyone, and so my mother always had to hang on to me tightly after meetings, or she would find me a block down the street shaking hands with people.

I enjoyed my life and all the attention. I was the only grandchild on both sides of the family and the only child on the team. I enjoyed singing in front of people, even though I got bored during some of the messages and thought the invitations were too long.

We traveled a lot, met hundreds of people, and knew all the bigwigs in the Christian world. I didn't even know there were any other kind of important people. However, as time went by my father began to get tired of radio, radio, and more radio. He was beginning to not care if he ever saw another microphone as long as he lived. It was also apparent that he would always be second in responsibility to his father, and he was ready for something he could direct. It was not an easy decision to leave something he had been a part of for so long, but he knew he had to make the break and get out.

This was during the very beginning days of Youth For Christ, (Y.F.C.), a new, exciting, and fast-moving organization that was catching on all over the country.

Bob Pierce (who later founded World Vision International) asked my dad to move to the West

Coast and travel full-time for Y.F.C. as a special speaker, and so we did. We joined the Pierces in Seattle, Washington. My mother's Aunt Bess went with us and stayed with me while my folks traveled from one end of the country to the other in Youth For Christ rallies, conventions, and evangelistic meetings.

Let me insert that as sick of radio as my dad was, it wasn't long until he started making transcriptions and sending them back to Pennsylvania. The "Bit of Heaven Ministry" was with us for a long time.

After about six months we moved again, this time to Portland, Oregon, where Frank Phillips was directing Youth For Christ—one of the largest in the country. That became our headquarters, and the traveling continued.

I traveled with my parents sometimes, and when possible I sang and took special parts in the programs. However, by now I had started school and was making a dramatic discovery. There was a whole other world out there. There was a world full of boys and girls who didn't go to church, who had never heard a gospel song, who had never seen an altar call. I was fascinated by the fact that some families played baseball and went camping on the weekends. And I was *really* fascinated by the fact that they seemed to be happy and well adjusted without a Christian world. I began to ask myself this question: Who got the better deal, them or me? I never asked aloud, however.

There was a group of people in Portland who wanted to start a church, and they asked my father to help them by being their pastor. After all the years of traveling, being more settled sounded good, and so my father founded the Evangel Baptist Church, which started out in a lodge hall with about twenty people. My grandfather died about this time, and my grandmother dissolved the Lehman ministry and moved to Portland together with my dad's sister Dorothy.

I thought my grandmother was terrific. She was eccentric, dramatic, and a great speaker with a flare for the unusual, which I eventually found out was unreality. She liked me too. I was a chip off her son. I liked the platform, and she soon became *my* coach, too. I remember one time in particular when I was the speaker—at five years of age—for the Women's Temperance Union League convention. She wrote the speech, and it was long. I memorized it, and then the drilling began. I stood in her living room and did it over and over until every inflection and gesture were perfectly placed. The speech was well delivered in front of several thousand people, and I got a new pair of roller skates as a reward.

My father's church grew rapidly, and I began to find out that there wasn't much difference between being an evangelist's kid and being a pastor's kid. My folks didn't travel as much, but they were gone a lot. Even then I realized the pressure that church society puts on its own people. That standard of judging whether a pastor and his wife are what they ought to be by how many church meetings they attend each week, and that ever-present knowledge that you have to be what people think you ought to be, make it difficult to show how you really feel or say what you want to say. There were very few people with whom my folks really let down their hair. Those few people were people just like them, in the same kind of work, who didn't have that opportunity very often either.

My only sister was born when I was seven. I didn't like the idea, or her very much for that matter. I had been the only child and the attention-getter for a long time. As the years went by, the age difference proved to be a hindrance to our being close, and the fact that our personalities were as different as night and day didn't help.

I had started piano lessons when I was four-and-a-half, which at that time I liked. I did well in school, rode a bike, and played with kids my own age. But even then I felt that other kids thought I was different. I sang in front of people. I took part in programs. I talked about wanting to grow up to be a performer. This might not have been unusual in an entertainer's family, but in a preacher's family thirty years ago it didn't sound right. People thought it was a phase—something I would grow out of.

Already I was a kid who was in trouble a lot. I was vividly aware of this and used to wonder if other kids did wrong things as often as I did. Obedience was not one of my virtues, and I have always talked too much ever since I can remember. I had a tendency to be bad even when I wanted to be good. I tried so hard sometimes that I ended up in worse trouble. Making some kind of spiritual decision (which in my experience usually meant a publicly made decision) seemed like the best way to show people I was trying—that I wasn't all bad. I never felt unloved, but even as young as I was, I began to feel out of place.

When I was seven years old, following one of my father's messages, I went forward to "make a decision" to accept Jesus Christ as my personal Savior. As I look back, a combination of emotion and the need to do what was expected and get approval was the motivation. Everyone was pleased, and shortly after that my father also baptized me.

My father was gone a lot and when he was home, he spent most of his time in his study. He wasn't much for chit-chat. Logically, because he had such an unusual childhood, he didn't know what to do with children most of the time. Rather than deal with a skinned knee or hurt feelings, he studied—undisturbed.

My father and I could communicate in one area—the area of creativity. Therefore, having his approval of my performances became very important. I idolized his mind, his abilities, and his creativity. I wanted to be just like him. He has always loved me very deeply. I often felt that he didn't know how to show me. The little ways that come so automatically to most people were very hard for him. Now, as an adult, I know why. I wish I had known then.

The Evangel Baptist Church was averaging 500 in attendance each Sunday in 1951 when my dad accepted a call to move to Grand Rapids, Michigan, to pastor the Calvary Undenominational

Church. I was nine; my sister Cheri was two. As I look back, this move brought about more changes in my life than any other one move.

Grand Rapids was a little world all its own.

CHAPTER 3

THE TEEN-AGE MISFIT GAINS WEIGHT

On the first Sunday in Grand Rapids, as we turned into the church parking lot, a car pulled in just in front of us, driven by a little white-haired man who was smoking a big cigar.

I was shocked and assumed that he had come only to leave someone off. After all, I knew one couldn't be a Christian or a member of my father's church and smoke a cigar at the same time.

After pointing him out and making sure to ask if my assumptions were correct, my father informed me that in Grand Rapids a lot of men in the church smoked cigars—but here Christians didn't buy or read Sunday newspapers. That didn't make much sense to me. My nine-year-old mind couldn't understand different sets of rules for different groups of Christians, a reality I would keep bumping into for the rest of my life.

My understanding of this is a lot better today, but I'm not so sure it makes much more sense now than it did then.

The church in Grand Rapids was bigger, and I liked that. It seemed to make us all more important. We settled into the parsonage, and I enrolled in a new school, acquired a new Sunday school teacher, and met a new set of peers. Another segment of life began.

What happened to me in the next few years was not all pleasant. I can't even explain a lot of it very well. But I do know that working through the impressions, attitudes, and patterns that were established between the time I was nine and seventeen has been difficult. In fact, they still creep up on me at times.

It wasn't long after we moved that I auditioned to be a soloist with the Children's Bible Hour, a weekly radio program that is still having an effective ministry among young children all across the country. I was selected, and until I left the broadcast at age fourteen, I did solo work and joined a little boy named Dick in duets and sang in the choir. My sister also joined the program less than a year later, at the age of three, as one of the tiny tots.

My experience and training through this program have proven to be invaluable ever since. Although I didn't appreciate it then, I have been grateful for it many times since.

Bertha T. Shooks, director of the program and known to everyone as "Aunt B," was quite a lady. I loved her, hated her, respected her, hugged her, and wanted to beat her up all at the same time.

She was hard on me and didn't think my stunts or temper tantrums were cute. I spent a great deal of time in her office. I had a way of making everything difficult. During one rehearsal I crawled under the piano and refused to come out. But she loved me and was one of those few people who believed with all her heart that even though you couldn't see it, there was something in me worth fighting for, a potential that someday I would recognize and that someday God would use.

A few months ago I saw "Aunt B" at a Children's Bible Hour Thirty-fifth Anniversary banquet. She couldn't see very well and gave me more than one hug to check out how thin I was, and she whispered in my ear, "You know, I've always held a special place in my heart for you." Somehow I always knew that, even though I gave her a hard time.

It was shortly after our move to Grand Rapids that I began to gain weight. At first everyone thought it was a "pleasingly plump" stage, but I grew out of that before long and graduated to being fat.

Everything about me seemed to turn from bad to worse in those same few years. My temper got worse, uncontrollable at times. My lying increased, and my inability to get along with my own peer group became more evident. My mood was always either very high or very low. I talked more and more and louder and louder. People constantly pointed out my bad points. What they didn't know was that I was always more aware of them than they were. I began to dislike myself.

Sure, everyone thought I was talented or gifted or creative or whatever word you want to use. However, they didn't really know what to do with that part of me. And besides, I was getting so heavy. I longed for a sentence that didn't have an "if" or a "but" in it, such as:

"You are a born leader. Now *if* you'd just not go so far overboard."

"You've got so much talent, *if* you just had some discipline to go with it."

"There's no limit to what you could do *if* you'd just lose weight."

"You want people to like you. You want boys to like you. You want to be invited places. *But* until you take that weight off, you'll never get those opportunities."

A lot of these things were true. Many of these people were right, but I wanted them just once in a while to say:

"You're terrific! I like you for what you are . . . just the way you are."

My mother and I began to have some severe problems. She is a beautiful lady and always has been. She is gracious, soft-spoken, and well-liked. She dresses well and does the right thing at the right time. Yet she didn't know exactly what to do with me.

My weight and overpowering personality irritated her and, at times, embarrassed her. I am sure that what she always dreamed about in a daughter and what she got were two different things.

Every time we went shopping for clothes we ended up in an argument. I wanted to dress like all the other girls, but my shape said no. Circular quilted skirts, sissy blouses, and lots of crinolines were in style, but I looked like a walking pickle barrel in that kind of thing. Everything I tried on either didn't fit or made me look too big. My mother would sit in the fitting room with a disgusted look on her face until she couldn't hold back any longer. Then she'd finally say, "Until you lose weight, you are not going to look good in anything." I'd retort, "Is the way a person looks the only thing that's important to anybody?" And away we'd go. I wish I had a nickel for every time we fought over excess pounds.

Piano lessons were still a weekly routine—and now a headache for the most part. As is true with most children taking music lessons, getting me to practice was a hassle. I'm sure that my parents were tempted many times to just let me quit . . . it would have been a lot easier. My mother and father both spent many hours making sure that the time was put in, and put in effectively. My response was less than appreciative. I did such things as hitting the piano, pounding the keys, telling them I hated them, and reiterating that I didn't want to play the piano at all.

I was convinced at that ripe old age of thirteen that talent was terrific, but work and discipline were needless. I wanted to perform, but I didn't want to practice, and I wouldn't listen to anyone who tried to tell me it doesn't work that way.

That is a lesson I eventually learned, but I learned it the hard way. I am thankful my parents had the ability to look beyond the daily hassle to the point when I would appreciate the fact that I could really play the piano. My father says to this day that he enjoys my playing above and beyond any concert artist in the world, not because I play that well, but because he invested a great deal more time and money in me than in all those others.

I wanted to direct Broadway musicals, be an actress, write poetry, travel with a musical group.

My fondest memories of Grand Rapids were the opportunities I had to meet all the musicians and speakers who came to our church, stayed in our home, and ate at our table. Because of the size of our church there were a lot of them—all the big names in evangelistic and gospel-music circles. I would sit in the front row and never take my eyes off them, noticing how they were dressed, watching every move they made, and listening to every note of their music. I wanted to be just like them when I grew up.

The kids at school were beginning to fall apart over a new rock star named Elvis Presley, but not I. These other people were my idols, the stars of my world. To be able to sit beside them at the table, to carry their music, and to hang up their coats were a real privilege.

The Youth For Christ convention held every year at Winona Lake, Indiana, was one of the largest conventions in the country. During those years my father was a frequent speaker and the family usually went along. I don't ever remember being as excited as I was during those weeks—all the greatest names in gospel music, choirs of 200 to 300 people, brass instruments, a big stage with curtains and back drops, and people everywhere. I loved crowds and noise and lots of action (I still do, but not quite as frequently).

One day I was stopped on the grounds of Winona Lake and was asked to deliver a music manuscript to a certain room in one of the hotels up the hill. I willingly did so with a feeling of great importance. I walked into the hotel and looked for the ballroom. It was quiet, and as I pushed open the door to the ballroom I saw no one in the immense room with its high ceilings but Ralph Carmichael, sitting behind a large table. My knees shook and my heart pounded just to think that I was there all alone with such a man. I walked over, handed the music to him, and noticed that he was writing music without a piano or an instrument of any kind. He wasn't even humming to himself.

This was the first time I realized that there were people who actually heard the music in their heads and knew what notes to put on paper. I stood and stared, and even though I have met many people since who do this all the time, I will never forget the impact that had on me. This man was a genius, and he was also the music director for the convention. He directed the choir I was singing in, and there I was standing right beside him!

It was interesting to me that during that week I heard more than one conversation among the leaders of the convention that touched upon the fact that they didn't really feel Ralph Carmichael would be able to stay alive in the Christian world. He was too progressive; his music sounded too secular, and most places weren't ready for or-chestra and brass backgrounds.

They were right. He had a hard time for many years. But I would like to insert that whether you like their music or not, Ralph Carmichael and John Peterson, another Christian musician, did more to change the world of gospel music than any other two people.

If they had not fought the criticism and the tradi-tion, young people would not be enjoying the gos-pel music they are today. I am personally grateful to them both.

My father put on a full dramatic pageant at Winona Lake one year. I was in it. I played the part of a postage stamp. I won't go into the explanation of that, but even though the part may seem strange, to me it was "Broadway."

We rented a truck to take all the props from Grand Rapids to the convention. We had rehear-sals and a large cast and music and special light-ing. The thing I liked most was the backstage pandemonium. I loved the hectic excitement and all the last-minute details. I felt that was where I belonged. My father was terrific and still the one I wanted to be like, particularly at times like this.

Sunday school became a drag. Church became a time to exchange wallets and write notes. Young people's meetings were dull and uninteresting, with such highlights as Bible drills and panel dis-cussions on why we shouldn't dance or go to movies.

Occasionally, I would be asked to be in charge

of a meeting. I would immediately start planning a production, writing a script, and enlisting people to take a part in the program. Most people thought I was a little strange, and admittedly I did go way overboard at times. But I honestly felt there had to be something better than what we usually did!

A couple of times I got stopped in midstream, and my plans were nipped in the bud. No one but Grandma Lehman, who had now moved to Grand Rapids, felt the church was the place for "all that theater stuff," and besides, no one wanted to encourage my worldly tendencies.

Junior high was a difficult time. Social pressure and peer acceptance were all important. Being the fattest girl around was painful.

I went to a big public school with grades seven through twelve in one building. By this time I was involved in Youth For Christ, singing in an ensemble, and attending my school Y.F.C. Bible club, which was the only school club or extracurricular activity I belonged to. I was still on the Children's Bible Hour, which involved two rehearsals each week, taping on Saturday morning, and traveling frequently on weekends with the other kids on the program to put on special programs in churches all over the state of Michigan.

Plus, of course, we were in church Wednesday nights, all day Sunday, Monday nights for Pioneer Girls (the Christian version of Girl Scouts), and any other time there were special meetings. I was busy, indeed smothered, and more unhappy than ever before.

I knew for sure now that there was another world out there—one with more exciting music, one without so many rules, one that went to the theater, sang secular music, wasn't afraid of rhythm, and one that I wanted to be a part of.

Food was becoming more and more important to me. I didn't want to be fat, but the more lonely I felt because I was fat, the more I ate. Chocolate was my number one weakness. I began to steal money regularly from my parents in order to buy four or five candy bars on the way home from school every day. They always found out and accused me, but I would never admit to taking the money and there would be a big fight.

Getting punished for things never seemed to make any difference to me. The pleasure of the moment was always worth whatever I thought I would have to face, a pattern that included not only food but also any pleasure I thought was worth the risk.

The only things I ever shoplifted were candy bars—five of them—when I was eleven years old. I ate them all in five minutes so there wouldn't be any evidence. However, the real evidence hung on for twenty-five years and still stares at me from the extra skin left between my knees and my waist.

My whole family had a tendency to gain weight, but none of them let it get out of hand as I did. My mother made a special effort to serve meals that would help us, and if my eating had stopped at the table, I might not have a story to tell.

My folks also entertained guests a lot, and therefore there were many times when there were fancy goodies around, either left over from the night before or bought to serve the next scheduled crowd.

After my nutritious meal, when the folks were gone or busy upstairs, I attacked the deadly delights. I was always under the delusion that no one would ever miss two tablespoons of icing from around the bottom of a cake or one small scoop of ice cream that anyone could have taken.

In my naive days, I never thought it was possible for someone to notice the absence of one piece of coffee cake, one sliver of pie, or three small pieces out of a complete box of candy. It would make me so mad when someone found out.

As time went by, I became braver, even though I knew it meant trouble. I couldn't stop with one piece or one slice; I would nibble until the damage done to the party fare was obvious even to me. Needless to say, my mother was not always delighted when, to her surprise, portions of what she had planned to serve were missing.

The prize thing I did was to eat all the ice cream in the carton and put the carton back in the freezer, thinking that when my mother looked at it everything would look the same. However, when she got ready to serve pie a la mode to our waiting guests and found the carton empty, her reaction was predictable. She would never bring up my eating sprees in front of our guests, but after they left she and I would go to blows.

Soon, having run out of ideas of how to get

through to me, she had to hide anything that was loaded with calories or that she wanted to protect for the next twenty-four hours.

She tried, and she did a pretty good job, but whenever I was alone in the house, the scavenger hunt would begin. I would find almond coffee cake under hats in hat boxes, one lonely box of candy between the layers of tablecloths in the buffet, half of a cake camouflaged in the garage.

I'm sure my parents had many a late night discussion about my eating habits, which were progressively getting worse. When the subject was brought up to me, however, I exploded.

My parents could always tell where I had been or what I had been doing. There were candy bar wrappers in the night stand, candy kiss papers in my underwear drawer, doughnut bags in my purse, and milkshake containers in the closet.

My mother took me to the doctor many times. The doctors always had a nice little talk with me about how heavy I was, what it was doing to my body, and how they could help me. I would always leave with a new diet, sometimes a prescription for pills, and a bad attitude toward doctors.

I would go on the diet—at home—for awhile. But soon the fact that I was eating behind everyone's back and throwing the pills into a drawer or on the closet floor would cause another blow-up and the end of another diet.

My grades got worse in school. My attitude about church was no longer well concealed. I didn't have any close friends, no boy friends like the other girls, and my emotional life kept everyone on the edge of his seat.

I even got thrown out of Pioneer Girls. (And remember, I was the pastor's daughter.)

I was so aware of the things I couldn't do, both because of the rules I lived under and now also because of my weight. The list of things I could do seemed very limited—mostly going to meetings and singing gospel music.

Even our family vacations for the most part consisted of going to Bible conferences for weeks at a time where my father spoke the whole time. Occasionally we would take a day on the way or on the way back for our leisure vacation. My father didn't know much about leisure. After a day's rest he paced a lot and seemed to feel guilty for not working.

I remember one time my father took me to a theater-in-the-round in a little resort area we drove through. What a marvelous experience it was—a musical, too. My father loved it as well as I did. He loved dramatics and poetry and music. Why did we all have to feel bad about enjoying these things occasionally?

Even though I was beginning to hate the Christian world I lived in, I wanted to be accepted by it. I wanted approval. I wanted people to know that I was good and that I didn't want to be bad. Spiritual approval was what I wanted most. I thought if all the people around me were convinced I was spiritual, they would like me, accept me, and approve of me.

Therefore, I made many spiritual decisions. I believe I dedicated my life to every mission field in the world at one time or another. I cried and repented and prayed and gave testimonies over and over again. They weren't *all* just for effect. Many times I felt that another decision would really help.

I have thrown myself across my bed hundreds of times in my life, angry at God for the way He had made me. Why was I fat? Why did I have all the wrong desires? Why was I interested in all the wrong things?

There were two facts I thought I knew for sure at this point: (1) There were certain kinds of personalities and certain kinds of ambitions that got the stamp of approval from Christian society, and I had neither. (2) No one would ever love me as I was. No one would want me, and I would never have any friends or opportunities to become what I wanted to be as long as I was fat.

My attitude was so bad and I had such a poor image of myself that many times I imagined that everyone was telling me what I had already come to believe about myself. But on the other hand, let me say that *in fact* that impression was clearly given to me in word and attitude by many of the people around me. Of course, they were all just trying to help.

I guess I finally set out to prove that everyone was wrong and that I was right. Someone, somewhere would love me just the way I was.

A few boys came along in junior high who were

nice to me—even dated me a time or two—but I always blew it.

I scared them to death!

When a girl wants a boy friend as badly as I did, and she has the aggressive personality I had, the relationship doesn't have a chance.

There was a boy named Bill who hung on longer than usual. I met him in school. He was Catholic. Needless to say, I didn't mention him at home for awhile.

When my glow of love became too bright to hide, I told my folks *I had a boyfriend!* The first question was not, "Is he nice?" or "Is he clean?" or "Is he from a nice family?" but "What church does he go to?"

I dodged the question for awhile, but made up a good, solid evangelical answer like Broadway Baptist or Third Presbyterian. I don't remember exactly now. Several months later, Bill walked me home from school. My mother invited him in for some refreshments. As the three of us were sitting at the kitchen table, Bill leaned forward to eat his ice cream and his St. Christopher medals fell through the opening in his shirt and clanged all over the table top. In 1956 no one except Roman Catholics wore medals—and so the end of the romance.

I had always been sneaky and deceitful, but at fourteen my real double life began—one that continued for many years.

This double life-style, I am convinced, was the main reason for the continued weight gain and the emotional destruction that followed. For years I went to sleep every night with a knot in the pit of my stomach, knowing that some day everything would blow up in my face.

Because I didn't have friends my own age, I hung around with older kids some of the time. When I was fourteen, one of my "friends" introduced me to a twenty-four-year-old guy who was the best friend of the fellow she was dating.

How flattered I was by his attention. I was willing to take any risk to be with him. I skipped school to see him and went out with him while I was supposed to be at Youth For Christ on Saturday nights. There is no doubt in my mind that this relationship was one of the most serious mistakes I ever made. My life, emotionally, sexually, and mentally, was never the same again.

In my immaturity I had proven everybody wrong. Somebody did want me just the way I was—fat—if only for a little while. I was too dumb to see that none of it was real, and too unwilling to realize that God had something better for me.

My parents were sensitive enough to know that some change had to be made, that I needed a creative outlet. I needed to be in stimulating surroundings with other talented kids who would give me stiff competition and help me develop my abilities.

We found out about a Christian high school that had a strong emphasis in music, writing, and speech, and I quickly agreed to go. I, too, thought that going away and getting my teeth into creative things would make all the difference in the world.

My folks took criticism from a lot of people who couldn't understand the wisdom of sending a fourteen-year-old away to a boarding school. There were also many people who felt parents only did this to get rid of children they couldn't handle.

Admittedly, I was a lot to handle in more ways than one. But that is not the reason I went away to school. I wanted to go. I felt a new place would surely solve some of my problems. It was my choice. And my parents, I'm sure, felt that this might be the "something" that would click with me and turn me around.

It was a beautiful school, one of very few boarding schools of its type. It combined the cultural and the spiritual—and definitely believed in the concept that a Christian young person should know how to dress and what spoon to use.

There were a lot of good things about the school, but I do feel the life-style was in some respects too removed from reality. I completed my remaining three years of high school there, worked in Bible conferences during the summers, and was graduated in 1960.

Those three years weren't any happier really. There were good times—moments when I felt like life wasn't such a hassle. But all in all, I was the same. There was one interesting difference, however. A certain percentage of the student body was made up of preachers' kids, missionaries' kids, and evangelists' kids. Some of them were also struggling with a lot of deep problems, but some of them seemed to be okay. They had a good attitude.

They really knew what they believed. When I looked at them, I knew for sure there was something wrong with me.

I had traveled all those miles and found myself in the same little world. Chapel every day. Church and concerts on the weekends. Bible conferences, dormitory prayer meetings, and mandatory personal morning devotions. There were even extra meetings thrown in when a good speaker dropped in on campus. I didn't care if I sat through another meeting as long as I lived.

The competition was good for me. I had always been one of the most talented kids around, but all of a sudden there were many who could outsing me, outplay me, outspeak me, and outstudy me.

My grades improved just from wanting to keep up with the key kids on campus, but grades weren't everything and I never was one of the "in" circle. A new place and new people had not made a new me. I was still too fat and not spiritual enough.

The school offered music and speech activities, but the opportunities went to those who exhibited a greater willingness to live up to the faculty's expectations. And while the good ones were learning their speeches, I was usually having a heart-to-heart talk with the housemother or sitting alone somewhere still wondering what was wrong with me.

My weight became more and more of a problem. Not many boys would date me; I was ashamed to be seen in a bathing suit, found it hard to run laps and play basketball with everyone else, and was in pain most of the time from the heavy girdle I wore and the nylons that cut my legs.

I wanted friends more than anything in the world. By this time I was so convinced I didn't deserve them and I would never have them that I didn't even know how to begin to make them. This still remains one of my hardest struggles.

I had one close friend in high school. I guess she was a close friend. I kept hoping she wasn't just being nice to me. Linda was beautiful. She had long dark hair, was well liked, well thought of at school, and was very active in speech and music activities. I never knew why she liked me, but she was the only person who gave me a feeling of acceptance.

Birthdays were special days in high school. On your birthday you always chose your best friend to bring your cake to your table during dinner. The whole student body sang as the cake bearer marched around the dining room. When my birthday came around, there was never any question who I would ask to carry my cake. I only had one friend. But when Linda's birthday came around, I would die inside for two or three weeks, knowing that she would probably ask one of her many other friends. She never disappointed me though, and she will never know how exciting it was for me to carry that cake to her table. It was my chance to say to all the other kids, "See, I have a friend, too."

Thanks, Linda.

By this time I was old enough to have definitely decided that the other world out there was a better place. I was reading (secretly, of course) about the teen-agers with hit records, parts in television shows, and lead parts on Broadway. And here I was learning Bible verses and all the words to all the stanzas of "A Mighty Fortress Is Our God." There was always the feeling of being pulled apart by wanting that other life while at the same time wanting acceptance in the only world I had ever lived in.

During my senior year I went on the last "real" diet I ever attempted until four years ago, and I did rather well. I used graduation as my goal and got down to a size 16 dress. I was so proud of myself and was even halfway confident in a bathing suit on our senior trip.

Being on a diet around teen-agers who eat hot dogs, cake, and candy bars is no easy thing, but I did well and graduation got closer. Along with this came a real desire to cooperate with the school directors and to show some improvement in my attitudes. I gave my senior piano recital and kept my grades high enough to be on the honor roll. Also, I had written for catalogs and entrance information from several Christian colleges that offered music and dramatic training.

When the junior/senior banquet time came around I was excited. The seating arrangements were always well planned by the faculty. They put couples together who were dating, and then the rest of the students were placed to their liking.

I was thinner; I was trying harder to be what they wanted me to be; my grades were good. All in all, I had improved. I wanted so badly to be seated by a good-looking boy. I had never been able to date the guys I wanted to date, and I remember lying in bed at night saying:

"God, just this once . . . just for me. Let me have one nice night. Make them seat me by someone I like."

The banquet night came, and in my new dress I walked around the beautifully decorated room looking for my place card. I was placed at a table with other girls.

I still remember that night. I remember how I ached inside, and I remember saying to myself, "Nobody cares how hard I tried. Even God couldn't let me have one nice evening." My conclusion was that I was still too fat and still had not reached the spiritual standard.

Another problem had to do with where I would go to college. When the faculty heard what schools I was interested in, I started having little private consultations. They went something like this:

"Karen, you know your weaknesses. If you go and study music and drama, it won't be long until you're in the secular world."

"You need to grow spiritually first. You need a couple of good years of Bible training before you get into those things."

"We would like to see you go to Bible school."

I didn't want to go to Bible school. I didn't want any more meetings. I felt guilty for not wanting to go and for not being spiritual. And again, even though I hated Christians at times, didn't want to be like them, and didn't like their pressure, I wanted their acceptance.

I sent for information, filled out an application and was accepted by a large, well-known Bible school.

When I announced my decision and in due time my acceptance, I received a strong pat on the back from the high school faculty and left with their knowing I had made a good decision and that I was finally on the right track. Their patience with me, so they thought, had paid off.

CHAPTER 4

ROUND PEG
IN A SQUARE HOLE

For several years after graduating from high school, if a stranger asked me where I went to college I would tell him Northwestern University where I majored in theater arts. It sounded good to me, but it wasn't true. I lasted two out of three years in Bible school.

The day after I arrived at Bible school (where my father was well known, by the way), I had my first interview with my counseling dean. After introductions and a few basic questions, we got down to the "nitty gritty." She asked, "What do you feel God wants you to do with your life?"

I answered honestly and sincerely, "I want to go into either radio and television or dramatics." Her facial response was less than warm and she asked, "Where do you plan to get that kind of training?" I explained that after Bible school I would probably transfer to a secular university that offered a degree in those fields. There was a long pause.

"Do you really feel that it would be pleasing to the Lord for a Christian young woman to pursue such a life's work?" she asked. My answer, of course, was yes. Her next phrase was a winner. "I

49

do pray that while you are here with us you will allow the Lord to work on your worldly tendencies."

Now, I admit that to me what God wanted for my life was not a priority and serving Him was not my goal, but her statement set the tone for the next two years and let me know on my second day that I was in a different city but in the same place I had always been.

From then on it was all of them (the faculty and deans) trying to do something about those same old worldly tendencies, while I was trying to prove something by tightly hanging on to them.

Meetings were again the mainstay of life. There were daily chapel devotions, dormitory and floor prayer meetings, missionary conferences, Bible conferences, etc. I was in a music course that helped break the routine some. And I did have some good times. I liked a lot of the music students and loved the times when we all got together, after practicing in the music building, to sing for hours. We would laugh until we ached and carry on like crazy people.

We also did some things that weren't too smart, like having water fights in the music building, both on and off the elevators. But these were the best hours, the times when I felt included and liked and happy.

The choir tours are also wonderful memories. I never wanted the tours to end. At this point in my life I could never get enough of living out of a suitcase, being in a different city every night, and always having something going on.

And believe it or not, there were also occasional meetings I enjoyed. Every once in a while a speaker would really ring my chimes—even disturbingly so—but I would push the few driven-home points out of my mind as quickly as possible.

And I got a part-time job writing continuity and singing in ensembles at a local radio station. I enjoyed that as well.

Again I was privileged to hear and work with many of the greatest musicians in Christian circles, and little did I realize that a number of my fellow classmates would be having a worldwide impact on those same circles a number of years later.

I had gained weight during the summer following high school and continued to gain at a fast rate from then on. I went from 180 to 270 pounds the two years I was in Bible school.

I didn't have any desire to sit through Bible courses, and I was even less motivated to study the Bible in my room. I made no attempt to grasp theology and eventually was caught cheating and flunked a course in that subject. I had missions class at 7:30 in the morning, and if I managed to stay awake at all, I found whatever I heard a joke. The only courses that interested me at all were music courses, and I really didn't do extremely well in those.

I ate eight to ten candy bars a day, never ate in the school dining room, and literally lived on chili dogs, chocolate malts, ice cream bars, and Coke.

I ate most of this junk in my room or in a stall in the bathroom or away from campus.

I would wait until no one was around the snack food machines and then get a day's supply at a time. I would never take the risk of buying candy bars in front of other people. After all, no one watches a fat person put money in one of those machines without making a remark to someone close at hand.

And I could carry all these goodies to my room without anyone knowing it. I'd stuff as much as I could in my purse and wear the rest up my sleeves, under my arms, or wherever my clothes would allow. A loose-leaf notebook works, too, if you hold it just right.

I also got on the laxative kick. I decided that if I would take four or five Feenamint tablets or five or six ExLax pills right after one of my binges, less damage would be done. It is a wonder, after years of doing that two or three times a week, that I have any insides left.

It was again very difficult to find clothes and I surely couldn't dress like everyone else. I was included in groups off and on, but was faced with the same old problems—no dates, no small groups of two, and no close friends.

It was during these two years that I made two decisions. First, that I would always be fat. I had put on so much weight and gotten so hooked on food that I knew I would never take it off. Second, I had the choice of either withdrawing and becoming a wall flower or building an image and a personality, using my weight as best I could.

I chose the latter, and from that day until that all-important day four years ago, I spent the majority of my time and effort building an image and being a self-contained, three-ring circus.

A character is what I was. I started trying to dress differently from everybody else. I assumed the attitude that I didn't need people, that I was self-sufficient. This was the best way I knew how to keep people from thinking I just didn't have any friends or that my weight kept me from entering into group activities. I worked at being funny. I learned how to make jokes about my weight and learned to laugh along with everybody else who thought those jokes were hilarious. I found (painfully) that I could flirt and no one took me seriously, and so I did. I found out how to enjoy those parts in a skit that are so much funnier if they're played by a fat person and even began volunteering for them.

I was really something. And somehow I found a security in all this, an attention I couldn't get any other way, and a little world that for the most part I thought was really me.

But I was so lonely. When the laughter stopped and the people walked away, it was just me. And in the hours I was forced to be all alone with me, I was still mad at God for making me that way. And I was still sick of meetings, and I still wanted out of the Christian world with all its rules and regulations, and I still wanted to be just like other people.

Between the dean of women, my counseling dean, and the housemother, I was indeed kept busy with personal appointments. It got so that I wanted to avoid my mailbox because there was always a slip informing me that someone again had found it necessary to see me.

Let me say that I deserved a lot of those sessions because I broke a good many rules, but because of my "worldly tendencies" I do think I was zeroed in on a little more carefully than some of my "spiritual" schoolmates.

I had the great honor of being called in for putting a rinse on my hair, for wearing fingernail polish, for having my bass fiddle in my room (which was interpreted to mean I was trying to make my room look like a beatnik joint), and for eating supper with another girl in a Jewish delicatessen that was located a little too close to some night clubs. I laugh about those things now, but there was nothing funny about them then. The more I got called in, the more convinced I was that whatever I would do, it would be wrong. Admittedly, I got to the point that I didn't care any more, and finally I did at times try to irritate them.

And every consultation would end with, "Karen, if you would just get your worldly tendencies straightened out, if you would just give your life over to the Lord, we wouldn't have all this trouble."

And there were times when I wondered if they were right, but I didn't want to do what they wanted me to do—surrender my life to the Lord. I didn't like their world and didn't want to live their life-style or talk their language. But their world was all I knew.

I was sneaking to movies, smoking off campus,

and continuing to live my double life. But even though I kept one foot in that other world I wanted so much, I always kept the other foot firmly planted in the world I knew best.

That other world scared me a little, and I hated myself for not being able to just get up, turn my back on my parents and the rest of Christian society, and walk away.

Down deep inside I always wondered if maybe there was some truth in all those Scripture verses and songs I had memorized over the years. What I did know for sure was that the Christian life was supposed to be an abundant life, giving peace and joy and direction and forgiveness of sins. I had spent nineteen years looking for those things, and I was still restless and dissatisfied and full of sin and guilt. I didn't know where I was going, what I wanted to do, or what place there really was for a fat, mixed-up preacher's kid. Following my natural pattern, I couldn't overlook all those people I had met who said they believed that Christ was everything and lived as though He didn't matter at all.

My need for love was very great. My realization that people had been right all these years about me and about my weight was stronger. I knew I would never date the fellows I really liked, and after all, my image was so overpowering by now that no one wanted to compete with that.

I did have one romance in Bible school with someone I didn't really want or love, but I felt I would have to adjust to it if I was to have any social life at all. He was really a nice guy, and he was good to me, but aside from the companionship and physical attention, my heart wasn't in it. We were even engaged for awhile, but I was bored with him; one day he dropped my bass fiddle, broke the bridge, and that was the last straw. I blew up and broke off the relationship.

I continued to build my image, to lose more and more interest in school, and to become more and more rebellious against the school and what it stood for.

A couple of times when I was really in trouble I did repent and cry and pray. But as time went by I didn't even do that anymore.

It used to scare me when I would remember how many times I had heard different preachers say that if you hardened your heart over and over again, the Lord wouldn't give you another chance to accept Him. I sometimes wondered if that was happening to me. I wouldn't have told anyone I thought about it, but I did from time to time.

One of my greatest questions for many years was why people were so quick to notice every wrong move I made but never seemed to notice my heartache and pain and struggle.

There were so few people who were willing to love me just the way I was. Most Christians know only how to love someone for what they can become.

During one of my school vacations, I mentioned out loud one day that a diet had crossed my mind. A good friend of my father who is a medical doctor heard about it. Logically he was very concerned about my weight. He talked to me, and because I was half interested and half not wanting to get into a hassle with an M.D. on obesity, I listened.

The outcome was that he personally bought and paid for a semester's supply of powdered Metrecal. I thought for a minute or two that it might work. He bought chocolate, which made it sound not quite so bad.

Back to school I went with two cases of Metrecal and a plastic shaker. This plan might have worked for a week at the most. It wasn't long until my room was known as the "milkshake pavillion." I supplied the dorm with in-between meals and before-bedtime specialties, all made with the Metrecal powder.

It wasn't long until I was eating exactly what I had been before, plus two or three milkshakes that I whipped up in my room. Of course, the worst part about it was having to look that doctor in the face the next time I went home. I was so embarrassed; I had failed again. I just knew what he must have thought of me. And my parents were embarrassed because he had spent so much money. I would have walked an extra mile every time I saw him, just to avoid talking to him.

Food became:

—my reward for doing something well,
—my comfort in disappointment,
—my sympathy in times of failure,
—my cure for boredom,
—my escape from all frustrations,

—my substitute for friends,
—my "something special" to look forward to,
   and
—my diversion from loneliness.

Food had become the most important thing in
life to me. I couldn't live without it. I'm sure it is
hard for someone who does not have the problem
to understand that overeating can be like al-
coholism. You become dependent on it even
though you realize what it is doing to you, even
though you hate what it makes you look like.

During my second year, everyone started talking about the junior/senior banquet and about the
fact that our class would have to come up with a
bigger and better program than ever before. I was
thrilled when an extremely talented young man
and I were chosen to be in charge. I did what you
might expect and immediately came up with
production-scale plans.

We worked hard for six months. I wrote the
script and the fellow wrote the music for a full-
fledged amateur Broadway musical. Before long
we had taken over a floor in an old building for the
construction of props. There were sewing machines running here and there throughout the
dormitory; there were several rehearsals a week,
and I was in my glory.

When I look at that script now, I laugh a lot. The
plot was so mild it almost wasn't there. The
dialogue was weak and the lyrics were trite, but at

the time it was terrific and far surpassed anything that had been attempted for that occasion before.

The day finally came to move everything to the school auditorium. The props were put in place, the ramp was built out over the audience for the entrance of the lead characters, and the cast put on their costumes for dress rehearsals. I sat in a chair about four rows back in that empty auditorium feeling every inch a director and watched my dream come true in color. I have had the opportunity to experience the thrill of seeing a theatrical production fall into place many times since then, but this one will always be the most exciting one to remember.

On the day of the performance, my mother and a friend of hers drove from Grand Rapids to view the finished product. They arrived very early and sneaked into the balcony in time to catch the warm-up show in which I was ironing out some last-minute wrinkles and checking everything out.

I was tired. I had worked day and night to put this thing together while keeping up with school. I hadn't gotten dressed for the banquet yet, and what my small private audience in the balcony saw was a disheveled but happy director. I was barefoot, having spent as many hours carrying my weight around as my feet could stand. I was dressed sloppily, and my hairstyle matched my attire very well. I was yelling at the top of my voice for a prop to be moved a little to the left and for the sound system to be checked one more time. I bounced my body on and off the stage a couple of times, avoiding the steps, and I freely wiped perspiration from my less than well-made-up face. Feeling good about the fact that everything was working, I went to the dorm to change and take a deep breath.

As the audience filed into the auditorium, they were overwhelmed by the props and preparations that had been made. As soon as the program was off and running, I paced in the back lobby, sticking my head in occasionally to see if all was going well.

The evening proceeded without any major disasters, and at the end the response was exciting. As the people left, I waited for some comment from the deans and faculty members. There were none. It had been suggested that this kind of secular-type production not be praised. After all, they didn't want to encourage young people to go into this sort of thing.

And when I met my mother in the back lobby, she was quick to precede any compliments with her disappointment in the way I had looked and acted earlier in the evening. After all, I would never get any boy friends that way.

As a result of that evening, there was a new policy at the school: no more secular programs. This one had been done too well.

For weeks afterwards, I occasionally would find a little note in my mailbox from a faculty member who thought the program was terrific.

But again I was bad—bad even for doing a good job. I felt guilty for doing something right and doing it well.

At the end of two years I beat the school to the punch. I took in a yellow departure slip before they could give me a pink one. I quit. My father was hurt, I am sure. I don't think he ever thought of himself as having a kid who would drop out of school. The trip home in the car was very quiet.

I didn't have any idea what I was going to do. I stayed home for the summer, worked for my dad some, and ate. In the fall we had a missionary conference at the church. One of the speakers was representing a missionary radio station. In a discussion around the dinner table one night he said the station was in bad need of pianists. I was available and certainly liked the idea of living in another country for awhile. Three weeks later I arrived in South America.

The first thing I discovered as soon as I got off the plane was that the Latins liked fat women, and I immediately thought about spending the rest of my life there. I was driven to the mission compound and shown to my apartment. Needless to say, it was not Park Avenue. I was there for a year and a half.

There is no doubt that I learned more about music during that time than in all the rest of my life put together. At first I just played the piano, but later I had the opportunity to sing and direct music, which was what I liked best. I learned to write choir arrangements, quartette and trio arrangements, and even some brass and string accompaniments.

I didn't speak a word of Spanish when I went and not a whole lot when I came back, but making myself understood was not the greatest problem I faced.

Of course, the thousands of miles I had traveled didn't separate me from my deepest problems. I found myself again in a little Christian world with 6:30 A.M. prayer meetings, Sunday services, special speakers, and conferences. I was the youngest person on the large staff, which made it difficult. The people nearest my age were quite a bit older and not really interested in what I wanted to do. I was definitely in the prime dating age and was told not to date any nationals. This would have been much easier to swallow had there been some Americans in my age bracket. I also questioned how it was possible to genuinely love people you so separated yourselves from.

And I was still fat. Even though the Latins liked it, the Americans I lived and worked with were really not much different from those at home.

While I was there, I met a wonderful family. They had three children, and the oldest had just gone to the States to college. They became my family while I was there and the only stabilizing force in my life during those months.

I don't know how many meals I ate with them or how many hours I bent their ears, but I want them to know it was worth it. We had a blow-up here and there, and they let me have it. One time in particular I was feeling sorry for myself—rationalizing why I was fat—pointing out every hypocrite in the world, and telling the mother of this family how awful the world was.

Well, let me tell you, I got it both barrels. I was told it was time I realized I had created a lot of my own problems. I was the one who was fat, and no one was going to have any sympathy for me. I was going to have to do something about it.

Oh, how I wish I would have been in the habit of listening to people. She was right. I lost control; I think I even threw something and slammed the door and left. I later cried and apologized and was forgiven.

These people didn't nag me or try to counsel me every chance they got. In fact, instead they showed me love and friendship and acceptance. I know they saw my restlessness and my pain. I know they knew my life wasn't what it ought to be. I suppose they even knew I was playing around with fire a lot of the time, but their door was always open, and on birthdays and Christmas there was a place for me and presents to open.

They didn't say much, but they hung on to me.

As you might expect, I fell in love with a Latin. Believe me, it wasn't for spite or to purposely break the rules; it was just me again.

He was handsome, intelligent, well dressed, and a medical student working his way through school as an evening radio announcer. After all those years of not having the chance to date the cream of the crop, how could I turn down such an opportunity?

This man made me feel like I was the only person in the world, a talent I'm sure he had acquired through vast experience. But I didn't have my eyes open far enough to see that. I fell hard and was willing to live a complicated double life to take advantage of what I knew was true love.

Again the sneaking and the lying and the planning inflated the ever-present knot in the pit of my stomach, but as I saw it, it was all worth it for him. I was really proving the world wrong this time. Someone really did love me.

This man was not a Christian and certainly did not live in a Christian world. Except for the few hours he worked at the radio station, he was definitely a part of that other world I had always wanted, and being with him showed me only the good parts of that world. He was exciting and took me to wonderful places and showed me a good time. I liked that world more than ever.

We eventually were found out. No one ever realized exactly what was going on, but the fact that I was seeing him finally hit the head man's desk. Needless to say, I was called in. I was given a choice: break it off or go home. Well, I didn't want to leave him, so I promised to call it quits.

Actually, we just played it low key for awhile, but the relationship never dissolved. In fact, when I finally left to return to the States, our wedding date was set and he was going to finish his education in the States.

I had thought so many times I would never find a place, a group of people, or a job where I would fit in the Christian world, where I would feel comfortable. If I married this man, I wouldn't have to walk away from the Christian world all alone. I would have him beside me. He would take me out of one world and into another and I would be happy.

My sister came to visit me a few weeks before I went home. It was the first time we had spent that much time alone, and because she was getting older, we began to be friends for the first time.

I left South America with wedding plans, my sister, and a big apprehension as to how my folks would adjust to a Latin, non-Christian son-in-law.

Well, I told them he *was* a Christian. That was the easiest way to handle that part. And after they gave me all the typical arguments on the nationality difference, they accepted the idea fairly well. I was twenty-one years old and at this point they knew me well enough to know I would do what I wanted to do anyway. I'm sure my folks thought maybe—just maybe—I would take some weight off for the wedding.

I wondered, never audibly, what my husband-to-be would think of his wife after he was in the States for awhile. I imagined that after he learned our culture, he, too, would think I was ugly. But even that thought didn't change the fact that I knew I couldn't do anything about it. The habit of eating had too strong a hold on me. I would never break it.

I would just have to take the risk of facing the future as it came. I got a job in a radio station and started to make wedding plans.

And I ate. I was now eating a dozen doughnuts at a time each day, in addition to candy bars and three meals a day.

CHAPTER 5

A FLING WITH THE WORLD

On the plane coming home from South America I did a lot of thinking about that other world. I wanted to be a success. I wanted to amount to something. I was tired of living a double life. I was smart enough to know I couldn't live in both worlds and succeed at anything.

In my estimation there was no way I would ever fit into the Christian world. My attitude and the years of being told I had never met the standards had convinced me of that. I wanted to get married and get out. I wanted to love, and I wanted my freedom. Most of all, I wanted peace.

One of the things that had bothered me most in recent years was the status of some of my childhood idols. Some of those people I had watched so carefully and wanted to be just like had fallen from their pedestals.

Christian people are always so quick to remind their own to keep their eyes on the Lord, not on people. I'm not saying that's not good advice, but when you are a teen-ager or even a young adult, and you are not a Christian, it doesn't work.

In fact, *most Christians* spend a lot of time

watching other people. As a young person, I really did expect the people who were in full-time Christian work—in meetings all the time—to live everything they preached.

Now there were many who did, but those weren't the ones I remembered. Being in the evangelistic world, working around Christian leaders, and having a preacher father also exposed me to the people who knew everything that was going on behind the scenes.

During these very crucial months of my life, I saw a few more fall. Among them were several who had been extremely important to me. I was cynical anyway, and at this point because of my one-sided focus, I decided there wasn't anybody who lived what he said. As a result, there wasn't much validity to Christianity in my mind.

The bridesmaid dresses were made, the church was reserved, the cake had been ordered, and my mother's friends and mine had both given me wedding showers. I was excited, read his letters over and over again, and could hardly wait until my handsome fiance arrived so I could show him off.

But suddenly the letters came less frequently, and finally a telegram arrived that simply said he wasn't coming. I have never seen him nor heard from him since.

How thankful I am to the Lord for protecting me even when I didn't want to be protected. That marriage would have been the disaster of the ages.

I wanted to crawl into a hole and never come out, I was so embarrassed. My room was piled with wedding gifts and all I had to go with them was a stack of love letters, a small collection of South American stamps, and one black and white photograph of the man who said he loved me. But he didn't want this fat, aggressive girl either. I was so hurt. I figured that everybody would think I had made him up or that I had wanted to get married so badly that I had misunderstood his intentions, or that I had scared him off as I had so many others.

I lived through it, probably without revealing to anyone the degree of pain and rejection I felt, but I came out of my depression with a couple of firm resolutions. One—I would never let myself be hurt again. I would protect myself. I would expect rejection and learn to live with it. This one decision that I learned to live by, and which finally became a part of me, was what several years later almost ruined my marriage. For a long time I didn't realize how ingrained this pattern had become. I am still going through the undoing of it.

The second decision was to get out of my little Christian world once and for all. I wanted to run away from everybody and everything. Maybe I would fit in that other world. I had to try. I wasn't happy where I was.

I got an offer to work in a radio station in Houston, Texas, and I took it. I piled everything I owned, and me, into my small brown Corvair Monza and headed out from the parsonage across country. I can remember my thoughts as I drove those many miles all alone. I felt free at last. I was finally going to have the life I had always wanted. I planned to have the life-style I had always dreamed about. I would look for the kind of friends that lived like I wanted to live, had my kind of interests, had connections with the kind of job I eventually wanted to have.

No one knew me in Houston. No one knew what my father did for a living. I didn't plan to look at another church, sit through another evangelistic meeting, or meet another Sunday school teacher.

My biggest goal in life was to do everything I had never been allowed to do without being found out and without being told how bad I was and without having to feel guilty. I looked forward to everything with great anticipation. And I was so proud of myself for making the break.

I arrived in that hot, humid territory with my clothes, a few left-over kitchen wedding gifts, and a new lease on life. I moved into a small unair-conditioned apartment and reported for work. I wrote copy, had a women's program, worked in programming, and got busy establishing my new life.

Right away I found out I was too fat and too broke to meet the people I had imagined myself with in this new world. I was too unknown and too foreign to secular music to meet the right people in the entertainment business. After facing that reality, I figured that the best thing to do was lower the standards for awhile, start at the bottom and work up. I just had to find my niche, that was all.

I found out about a small community theater group and went to see if perhaps there was a part available. They were grateful for any help they could get, and I began hanging around at nights to give assistance wherever it was needed. I liked the people. They spoke my language. They lived free, open, creative lives, and I began to feel at home. They were not exactly class, but it was a start. I began to learn a lot—like how to hold a lot of liquor after rehearsals, how to adapt my language so I sounded like one of them, and how to go to bars without feeling uncomfortable.

I loved it at first—couldn't get enough of the fun and freedom I was experiencing. But that filled just a few nights a week. The other nights were empty and lonely, and I hated to be alone.

From the day I started to work at that radio station, my work was always secondary to my thoughts about where I could find excitement and activity. For awhile it didn't show in my productivity and performance, only in my mind. My decision to start at the bottom and work hard to get to the top sounded good. But what really happened was I started at the bottom and worked down. The resulting deterioration of my total person is hard to write about.

My eating habits still controlled my life and at this point began to create a new kind of problem. I started eating every day in one of two crummy cafes. I got to know the managers and finally worked out a deal so that I could charge my meals and pay for them once every two weeks when I got paid. I ate three huge meals a day in one or the other of these two places and ordered stuff "to go" to take home late at night. Sometimes I sat for hours and drank coffee and ate desserts. I couldn't stop. When I got paid, I always paid my bills off in these two places first. I didn't want to lose my credit. After I paid for my food, I started having trouble paying my other bills. Pretty soon I had checks bouncing all over town and unpaid bills stacked here and there. On top of that, I never could discipline myself to write any amounts in my checkbook. (Sound like an alcoholic?)

Getting into this kind of mess and always living with people after me for money only added to my unhappiness. But I couldn't stop eating, and I always paid those bills first. I kept getting bigger, but I didn't have the money to buy new clothes, and so my wardrobe began to dwindle.

My life with the people at the theater and the few friends I had made was beginning to get ahold of me. The more I had, the more I wanted. It didn't make me happy, but it was some place to go, something to do. And there were people. I needed to be around people. I would do anything not to have to go home to that empty apartment. We used to go to one bar frequently. One night someone found out I could sing and asked me to get up and sing for the bombed crowd. I only had four or five songs in my secular repertoire (I didn't tell them that), but I went to the piano and sang the ones I knew. I was a hit with this motley crew, who probably would have applauded anyone. But I was flattered and thought for sure that this was the beginning of my secular career.

When I was by myself at night, I started going to that bar alone. I would order a drink and hope the manager would ask me to sing—but he never did. Sometimes I would sit there until one or two o'clock in the morning. I would finally get up, go home, and fall into bed. I would always try to go to sleep quickly so I wouldn't have to think about how lonely I was.

Those old feelings began to creep in again—those feelings that no one would ever want me, that no one would ever love me, that I would never be happy. I remembered those times in my life when I felt loved, if only for a little while, and wondered if maybe that wasn't the answer.

I began to look for love, for someone who would want me—maybe take me to dinner or to a movie. I needed someone to give me some attention, someone to whom I could be important.

I discovered that if you lower your standards far enough, if you're willing to ignore any sense of values, you can always find someone who is willing to do the same thing. The only problem is, they never take you out for a nice dinner or to a movie.

There is no need to go into detail, but I became someone I didn't even know. The standards got lower and lower. Being fat didn't help my marketability, and my life fell apart at the seams.

Between drinking and getting very little sleep, my life just started to all run together. My mind became possessed with sin. I didn't think about anything else.

Some of my new companions introduced me to pot—a way of getting a few more moments of happiness here and there. I got so low I didn't care how I looked. I was usually too tired to take a bath; I didn't care who I was with nor what I did, but I was seldom alone. How I went to work every day I will never know, but my productivity became almost nothing, and I couldn't think very well.

I didn't communicate at all with my parents during this time, except by phone when they would call out of desperation. Of course, the report they got was that all was going fine.

None of my "friends" knew what kind of background I had. They were never very interested, and if they asked I would tell them my dad was a preacher. Everyone would laugh and that would be the end of it. I never would admit that I believed in God or wanted anything to do with Him. But no matter how low I got or how far I ran, I knew He was real. I must have, for there were those nights when I would lie on my bed—dirty and confused—trying to go to sleep on sheets that hadn't been changed for weeks, and I would think, "God is going to get me for this." As hard as I tried to avoid it, I always felt guilty and always knew that this way of life wasn't the answer either.

Just let me insert that the greatest evidence I have today that God really had a purpose for my life was His protecting hand during this period of my life. The fact that I never got beat up by some drunk, or never got sick or pregnant or diseased is a miracle.

My "friends" finally began to disappear, and my reputation around town was shameful. I was in bad trouble financially. I knew my job was shaky, and I had found out I didn't fit in that world either. I had to get out of town. I gave myself a few days to pull myself together, and then I piled everything back into that little car, and with just a few dollars I started driving straight through—back to the parsonage in Grand Rapids, the only place I knew to go.

As I drove, I started telling myself I had better not lay my cards on the table about the mess I had gotten into. After all, I could put on a good performance and just pick up where I had left off.

I drove into the driveway, unloaded the boxes, told my folks that the job had just not been for me, and tried to act happy. My father had left the pastorate and had returned full time into radio and evangelistic meetings, but I took my place in the church choir and got back in with some of the faithful young adults in the church. Again, I assumed that double life I hated so much. I got a job at another radio station, which was filled with people who lived as I had in Houston, and I fell back into the same routine during certain hours, while I lived at the parsonage the other hours and went to church on Sundays.

My double life was now a lot harder to juggle. While in Houston I had formed some habits and the kind of life-style that was in far greater contrast to the Christian world than had been the case before.

I'm sure my parents weren't as dumb as I thought they were, and I wasn't as clever as I gave myself credit for. They knew many things were wrong, but I was a defensive, explosive twenty-four-year-old who wasn't about to seek their counsel. I don't think they knew how extensive my involvements were, but at this point nothing would have shocked them.

Nevertheless, I spent hours juggling my two worlds and couldn't look anyone in the eye. Every day I took the risk of everything blowing up in my face.

Emotionally there wasn't much left of me. I kept working at putting up a good front, but I was dying inside. I really didn't know what to do, but I knew I couldn't live the rest of my life in such turmoil. I had tried the Christian world for all those years, but I had never fit. I had never found all those things everybody else talked about: peace, joy, abundant life, direction, satisfaction. And I had tried the other world and had gone as far down the tubes as I could go. I didn't fit there either and had found none of the things I kept looking for. Neither world had the answers. What was I going to do?

I hated not only myself but God. If He had created me this way; if He had purposely given me all these conflicting emotions; if He enjoyed watching me struggle and fidget to find my place; if He was trying to prove something by letting me be in such turmoil and pain, then I didn't think He was at all what I had heard over and over that He was. However, at this point in my life God was preparing the way for something wonderful, only I didn't know it.

John W. Peterson—a well-known Christian composer—and Gospel Films were in the planning and writing stages of the first Christian musical to be put on film. I had known John Peterson for a long time. In fact, the first time I ever saw him was when he came from Chicago to sing at my father's church when I was twelve or thirteen years old. Since then, he had moved to Grand Rapids to be president of Singspiration (a Christian music publishing organization) and was attending the church my father had pastored.

For some reason, he liked the way I sang and thought I had potential. Before my move to Houston he had taken me to lunch because he was concerned about the fact that I was thinking about eventually going to Hollywood and trying to do night clubs. I'm sure he didn't think I heard a word he said, because I ignored it; but the fact that he took the time to be concerned impressed me more than he realized. After all, who was I to John Peterson? He tried very hard to help me understand that God could use me if I would let Him. He was one of those few people who saw beyond the outside all the way through to the real potential.

And even though I wasn't really interested in what God had for me, a couple of years after that meeting John Peterson still was. He and Billy Zeoli created a part for me in the film. And when I was at the point of wanting to die instead of going on in life all mixed up, I was offered the part of a girl named Kitty in "Worlds Apart." The picture looks antique now, but it played an important part in my life. John Peterson wrote a song for me called "Shepherd of Love" and took me to Hollywood to make the soundtrack.

Imagine! After all those years of wanting to "make it" as a singer, there I was in a professional recording studio with the R.C.A. recording orchestra recording, of all things, a gospel song!

I was given a script written by a man I had never met and was told to have my lines memorized by the time shooting began. As I read the script, I thought that this writer must have been following me around. The part I was to play was about a fat, funny girl who was always making people laugh. When things were serious, she was never around. At the end of the picture she was in an accident and put in a position where she couldn't be funny any longer and had to face what her need really was.

I didn't think about it a lot; I just memorized it. The day came for shooting to begin. I packed enough clothes to last six weeks and drove to Muskegon, Michigan, and checked into the Holiday Inn. The next day I reported to the studios to start work.

CHAPTER 6

An Important Step
in the Right Direction

Not long after I arrived at the studios of Gospel Films that first day, one of the staff people who had known my family and me for many years took me aside and said, "Some of the actors and crew that are coming in to make this picture aren't Christians. We're really depending on you to be a testimony. What a terrific opportunity to see some of these people come to know the Lord."

I died inside. Me a testimony? I almost wanted to laugh—or maybe cry. I didn't know which. I was probably more messed up than all the rest of them put together.

I met the actors and the crew. We went through wardrobe selections; I had some last-minute fittings, and then the shooting actually began. In addition, while certain scenes were being shot, we would have rehearsals for scenes coming up. I also had to spend time "lip-synching" (the singing parts were on tape, and we mouthed the words) my musical numbers, and I spent a lot of time working on the choreography for my Russian ballet number.

You read it right . . . a ballet number. It was a

comedy sequence, of course, but my body didn't laugh as I was put through the paces. I had to fall down, get up, lift my legs in the air, and twirl around over and over again, singing at the same time.

Needless to say, I wasn't a physical fitness expert, and every inch of me kept crying out in pain: "You're not ready for this." But I kept rehearsing and groaning, and for a couple of days I felt like someone had beat me to death.

I must tell you about the day I went to a local ballet store to buy my tights. That sequence itself should have been filmed. I walked in and told the sales lady I wanted a pair of black ballet tights and a pair of black ballet slippers. There was no change of expression on her face as she simply asked me, "What size does your little girl wear?" I didn't change *my* expression either as I answered, "They aren't for my little girl. They're for me, and I suppose I need the biggest size you have."

With this, her expression did change into bewilderment, and her speech changed into a sort of I-don't-know-what-to-do-now stutter.

Taking another quick glance at me, she said she would have to check the stock room, and with that disappeared to tell the other employees her predicament. Before long I heard snickers and subdued conversation, and of course, they all started finding some excuse to wander out and take a look at the fat lady waiting for her ballet tights. I could have explained, but that would have taken all the fun out of it.

Finally the saleslady reappeared with a small

box and held up a pair of tights that looked as if I might be able to wear them as elbow-length gloves, if at all. She told me it was the largest size they had and that they did stretch. I told her I would try them on, and while muffling her laughter, she took me to the dressing room.

I pushed and I pulled; I huffed and I puffed; and I finally got them up—to just above my knees. I opened the door of the dressing room, hopped out to where the lady was standing and said, "These fit just fine; I'll take them." I'll never forget how close she came to laughing right in my face. I took them off, paid for the tights and my slippers, and walked out. I'm sure they laughed the rest of the day and told the story to many a customer and friend.

I knew, of course, I wouldn't find my size and would have to cut the tights off and wear them as nylons, but they didn't know that. I'm sure they pictured me hopping through some weirdo's ballet class.

In addition to playing my part, I had the opportunity of directing the music for a couple of the crowd scenes where everyone had to lip-synch with the music we had taped in Hollywood. I enjoyed every minute of this and particularly the times when I got to stand on top of a ladder with a big sun hat on, shouting orders to a hundred young people on the Hope College campus in Holland, Michigan.

In one scene I had to fall backwards out of a boat into a lake. I discovered you don't just shoot a scene once when you're making a movie. You shoot it many times, each time from a different angle. I fell into the lake, changed clothes, put my hair back up under a straw hat, and fell out again—each time for a few more people who spotted the movie cameras and wanted to watch the action.

I was the only amateur actor with a lead part. All the others were pros from the West Coast. I felt like an amateur most of the time, but the others were wonderful to me. They helped me, encouraged me, and complimented me when I improved.

I was having the chance to do many of the things I had always wanted to do, and in the Christian world, too.

But as usual, I continued to blow it. I even took this marvelous opportunity and began to mess it up. What that man had said to me that first day kept haunting me. I felt pulled apart again between living like they wanted me to live and living with the same old habits and desires.

During the day I always made sure that I was in the restroom or just outside the building when everyone sat down to lunch. I was afraid someone would call on me to pray before the meal. I didn't want the Gospel Films people to think I didn't want to pray, but I didn't want the cast and crew to know I knew how to pray. My double life again. I said the right things and behaved a certain way while shooting or at the studio, and I lived the other way at night and on the weekends. Some of those weekends I even left town. Between the extra food I ate and a few airline tickets and hotel bills, I was spending my money as quickly as I made it.

I was fun and jovial, cooperative and energetic, but my heart ached for peace. I wanted to cry out for help, to admit there wasn't much left of me inside. I wanted to admit I was sick of being restless, sick of putting on an act, sick of life. But I couldn't. What would all those people who knew my family think? How would those people who had given me a chance react?

I wondered if God cared that I was down here, wandering around trying to find my place. I wondered if He knew how lonely and confused and dirty I felt. I wondered if He realized how shattering it was for me to find out, that even in doing the things I had wanted to do all my life, I was finding no satisfaction.

And then the day came when we were to shoot that scene where the fat girl I was portraying was put in a position where she couldn't be funny any longer, and she had to face her need. They took *off* the make-up this time, bound my head with bandages, and put me in a hospital bed. They adjusted the lighting, ran through the scene, and started the camera rolling.

The lead man, named Paul, walked through the door and said his lines, which in essence were telling me I needed Christ in my life. And I would come back with, "But would God take time for one lonely, mixed-up girl?"

The answer would follow, "Yes, Kitty. God

loves you. He cares what happens to you, to your life, to your talent."

And we would cut and do the scene again from another angle. We did it over and over, and I don't know exactly when it happened, but all of a sudden it wasn't Kitty asking that question anymore. It was me.

"But would God take time for one lonely, mixed-up girl?" Not an auditorium full, not a whole Sunday school class full, not a whole church full, but just me. Did He know I didn't want to live? Did He realize how desperately I needed Him?

And that answer kept coming back again and again, "Yes, He loves you. He cares what happens to you, to your life, to your talent."

As I lay there between takes with all the lights on me and all the people moving around me, it was as if I understood everything for the first time. For twenty-four years I had heard the gospel, had heard that God loved me, had heard that He could forgive my sins and give me a new life. But I had fought so hard to find an alternative—to prove He wasn't necessary in my life—that I almost forgot how to believe anything. And all the basic, simple truths of God's love and redeeming grace had somehow gotten smothered in my frustrated efforts to fit into a life-style called Christianity.

But all of a sudden it was clear. It was as if God were saying to me, "You don't have to meet any spiritual standards for Me to accept you. I'll take you just the way you are." What a relief it was. I felt that maybe I just might have a chance to start all over.

The crew thought I had become a terrific actress. I cried genuine tears all through the rest of the scene.

When we finished, we went right into taping the musical number, "Shepherd of Love," which I sang from the hospital bed. A lot of people have laughed at that scene, because it is a little unrealistic, but it will always be my song. When John Peterson wrote it many months before, I'm sure he didn't know how God would use it in my life. When I recorded it, I didn't ever imagine that it would become my testimony. But that day when I lip-synched it from that hospital bed, I meant it, and lived it, and cried all the way through it. You'll never convince me that God didn't give John Peterson special guidance in putting together these lyrics:

Shepherd of love, you knew I had lost my way.
Shepherd of love, you cared that I'd gone astray.
You sought and found me,
Placed around me, strong arms
to carry me home.
No foe can harm me or alarm me,
Never again will I roam.
Shepherd of love, Savior and Lord
and Guide
Shepherd of love, forever I'll stay
by your side.*

After we finished shooting I went back to my hotel room. On my knees by the bed I asked the Lord to come into my life, to forgive my sin, to give me a new life. I asked Him to somehow gather up all the pieces of my life I had left strewn all over the place and put me back together. I asked for His peace, for His direction in my life, and for some new and right desires. I told Him how sorry I was for the way I had fought Him and denied Him. I told Him how much I wanted to be different and how ashamed I was for the way I had lived.

On that hot day in August of 1965, I, Karen Lehman—preacher's kid, fat person, misfit—became a child of God. From that day on, I have never doubted my salvation, and I have always known that I had my own place in the kingdom of God.

I went to bed that night without a knot in the pit of my stomach and discovered how good it felt to feel clean. I didn't find it difficult, but instead rather exciting, to share my story with the staff of Gospel Films, and of course, they were thrilled.

At the end of the shooting schedule before everyone left, we all got together along with some of the Gospel Films board members and friends from the Muskegon area to watch some work prints. I had the privilege of sharing what God had done for me with these people whom I had lived so close to for many weeks. It was difficult, in view of the fact that they had all been a part of one side or the other of my double-life game up until the last week, but it was a big step for me to face them and tell them what had happened.

I must say how grateful I am to God for His patience, for His love, for His protecting hand during all those years. And I want to say thank you to my parents for all those years they hung on. You may have noticed that they haven't been mentioned much in the last couple of chapters. That tells you exactly how I treated them during that time. I ignored them. I couldn't tell them about my life, and so I didn't stay in touch. There were long periods when they never heard from me at all. No letters. No phone calls. No information. I know they lay awake many nights wondering where I was, what I was doing, and why I had to learn everything the hard way. I didn't want their life, their advice, or their help, and I told them so.

I am sure they wondered, as a lot of parents do, where they had gone wrong, why they had made so many mistakes (and they did make some), and I know they prayed that God would keep His hand on me and somehow bring me to the place where I would give Him my life. There was never a time that I questioned their love for me. There were times when I thought they didn't understand me nor accept me for what I was. But I knew they cared about me. Never once did they throw me out or tell me they couldn't have me living in the parsonage if I wasn't going to assume the "perfect" Christian life-style. I have told them I hated them, never wanted to see them again, and didn't want to be a part of their world. But they loved me and kept praying for me. And I want to say, "I love you, too, and thank you."

After the film was made and released, I traveled,

accompanying the film for the premiere showings in various cities around the country. I must admit I spent many hours in the back lobbies of churches and auditoriums. I got to the place where I had seen the picture enough to do me for a lifetime. After the film I would give my testimony and was thrilled over and over again when people accepted Christ as a result of the ministry of this film.

When you travel, funny things do happen occasionally, and I will never forget an incident that took place one night while I signed autographs in the back lobby of a high school auditorium. I had met a lot of people, shaken a lot of hands, and answered many questions about the picture, the actors, and, of course, about the cigarettes and the liquor bottles that had been used in some of the scenes. But one night I got one for which I didn't have an answer.

I saw this little man coming toward me. He had disheveled hair, a wrinkled suit, dandruff, and a big family Bible under his arm. I would have run if I could have, but I was stuck. He pushed his way in front of some other people, got up very close—in fact, too close—looked me in the eye and said, "Young lady, how do you have the nerve to get up and give your testimony and talk about what God has done for you after the audience has had to watch you throw your body around on the screen like that?"

My immediate impulse was to laugh, but I didn't. That Russian ballet comedy scene featuring the fat lady in her cut-off ballet tights was about as sensual as a box of oatmeal. I was usually gracious and answered all questions politely, but this one was a little too absurd for me. Impulsively, I leaned toward the little man, got right up in his face, and said in my most flirtatious voice, "Did you like it?" I'm sure he has never supported another Christian film.

While I was still traveling for Gospel Films, we got word that the film had won a number of awards from the National Evangelical Film Foundation, and the awards were to be presented at the annual awards festival in Philadelphia. I was thrilled when I was told I had won two of those awards, one for supporting actress of the year and one for female vocalist.

That night in Philadelphia was a very special night for me. To be recognized along with people like John W. Peterson; Billy Zeoli, president of Gospel Films; Al Kuhnle, vice president of Gospel Films; Lynn Borden, lead actress in "Worlds Apart"; and Dave Boyer, male vocalist of the year, was a great honor.

As a Christian with God's help I had gotten over some big hurdles. I knew now that I was a child of God, that He had a place for me and a purpose for me to fulfill. I wasn't quite sure what it was yet, but I wasn't wandering around aimlessly either. I had trusted God for salvation, for victory over some of the obvious deep sin in my life, but I hadn't learned yet to trust Him for everything. In fact, that's still hard sometimes. I had some problems that God hadn't helped me recognize yet, problems far deeper than I realized: cynicism, mistrust, selfishness, and, most of all, my eating habit.

As you read on, you're going to see that I've fallen on my face a lot as a child of God. I've struggled too much on my own instead of going to God for help. I've allowed myself to get away from daily communication with Him at times and have suffered and let depression take over as a result; but God and I have come a long way, and the most exciting part is yet to come.

One of the premiere showings of "Worlds Apart" was at Kansas City Youth For Christ. They showed it several nights in a row to a packed house, and I was there for a whole week. I did Bible clubs and luncheons and appeared with the film every night. While I was there, I was approached about moving to Kansas City to be the music director for the organization. It was a big operation with lots of opportunity and potential. The position was right down my alley, and after a lot of discussion and prayer I accepted.

I finished my traveling with Gospel Films, went home to Grand Rapids and packed for my move to a new place, a new job, and a new life. Just about everything would change for me in a matter of months.

CHAPTER 7

THE FAT CHRISTIAN

I pulled into the parking lot of Kansas City Youth For Christ on a hot and humid summer day in 1967. I was driving a 1962 Chevy Impala and pulling a U-Haul trailer that contained all my earthly possessions. All I owned consisted of music, old scripts, my mother's secondhand pots and pans, a set of dishes bought in anticipation of the defunct Latin wedding, and my grandmother's early version console television.

My wardrobe was also hanging across a pole in the back—thirty-five tent dresses, all in varying loud colors and designs. Of course, in addition, I had brought along my collection of shoes, purses, gloves and sun glasses, all coordinated very carefully to match each fat girl classic original.

Little did I know that I would stay in that city for seven years, while eating my way to 340 pounds.

I went to work immediately, and the routine I fell into along with the rest of the staff reminded me of those days my folks talked about many years ago. Everyone worked hard and long—six days a week, day and night, doing whatever had to be done.

This was the largest Youth For Christ organization in the country. They had their own auditorium, restaurant, office building, and camp. Dr. Al Metsker was its founder and director for twenty-eight years and he, along with his wife Vidy, put together a marvelous ministry. The organization is still going strong, and they have made a number of additions to their multi-faceted program.

Aside from the ministry of bringing young people to Christ, I was impressed with the opportunity they were giving gifted young people to develop their talents and gain performing experience.

As head of the music department, I was thrilled to be able to watch scared and awkward kids turn into effective and communicating Christian musicians. At any one time there would be 100 to 150 kids involved in the music program. You can imagine how many rehearsals and how much music it took to keep the thing moving. As always, the more hectic and busy it was, the more I loved it.

I had been there just long enough to get organized when I had to get everything together for summer camp. Because the new facilities weren't finished, the first summer camp was held, as it had been for several years, on the campus of John Brown University in Siloam Springs, Arkansas.

Planning the music for a week with 800 teenagers was a new challenge for me, but with boxes of materials and a week's supply of tent dresses, the other staff members and I piled into several cars and hit the road to be there two days early.

The day before the buses arrived we were busy setting up registration tables, going over schedules, and checking out the sound system. Because there were so few of us there, and everybody knew me, I ran around the whole day with big pink curlers in my hair. I did, however, wear a shocking pink flowered tent dress to match.

I had no idea that a few counselors were beginning to arrive, and among them was a twenty-seven-year-old single fellow from Wichita. As I was walking across the campus, I bumped into him. (Maybe I shouldn't put it that way. If I had bumped into him, he wouldn't be alive today!)

We exchanged a few words, and I directed him to where Al was and went on my way. I have since been informed that he had been warned about me a few months earlier. While in Wichita, a staff member had described me as loud, hard, domineering, and flamboyant, but extremely meticulous and right for my job. Even that, he tells me, didn't prepare him for the outfit nor the size, and in that first brief introduction he saw nothing of his ideal girl.

The next day I was standing beside him, watching the buses drive in. As the kids shouted at me from the windows, I impulsively ran over, grabbed this fellow's hand and yelled at the top of my voice, "Look, I've met my man. He's twenty-seven and single!" I didn't just say it once, but over and over as the buses drove by. I'm sure he must have wanted to crawl under a rock and die.

Larry grew up in Fredonia, a small town in southern Kansas, and was the youngest of eight

children. He, too, was from a strict Christian background, and to say he was staid and conservative is
an understatement. In comparison to me, he was
dead!

In the next few days we had opportunities to
talk, and he had a chance to watch me both on and
off the platform. Although I was everything that
normally turned him off, he began to see a part of
me that most people didn't see—the insecure,
lonely, "reaching out" me. He decided to be nice
to me for the week we were there. As he now says,
simply wanting to help me.

We became "the thing" on campus almost overnight. We were together almost constantly. We got
applause when we entered the cafeteria, whispers
when we sat together in the meetings, and throngs
of people when we tried to be alone. I played it to
the hilt, loved every minute of it, and hoped with
all my heart that it wasn't all a joke.

At the end of the week, instead of returning to
Wichita, Larry drove with the staff back to Kansas
City. He was scheduled to talk to Al Metsker about
becoming a full-time club director. I assumed that
I had something to do with his wanting to make
this move, but no such luck. Larry, too, was working through some personal inconsistencies and
was feeling pressured to enter full-time Christian
work. He felt that this was his chance to get out
from under these pressures and please others as
well. This, and not I, was the reason for his pursu-
ing this position.

Also, there was another girl, a girl he had broken
up with, who he still felt he would marry someday.

And she surely fit a lot more of his qualifications than I did. All the girls Larry had ever dated were conservative in just about every sense of the word. They were solid Christian society citizens, well thought of, and followed all the rules. They dressed conservatively, wore very little make-up, were submissive and much, much quieter.

Larry was asked to join the full-time staff and left for Wichita to resign his printing job, pack his clothes, and move. I could hardly wait until he came back, knowing that we really had something going. And he was packing, and hesitating, because he didn't know what to do about me. He was convinced it would all just blow over.

When Larry arrived, there was no way to make all those teen-agers believe he hadn't moved there to be with me. In their minds and remarks we were already engaged, happily married, and settled into a small, red brick house with a white picket fence. I thought it would be nice if it were all that simple.

We did see a lot of each other, and I was extremely happy. I was having a new experience. I was falling in love without a physical relationship. I didn't realize then that I would find out that I really didn't know how to love, to give myself unselfishly to someone. And Larry was having a new experience. I was a whole new world to him. He admits now that many of the things about me that at first went against his conservative Christian opinions began to fascinate him. I was impulsive and outwardly uninhibited. I had a flare for the unusual, the dramatic, the sensational, and believed wholeheartedly in the belly laugh. This twenty-seven-year-old man, that I don't think had ever laughed clear down to the soles of his feet, was being introduced to a flamboyant, spontaneous, exciting life he had never discovered.

He began to realize that he didn't have to be as proper and staid as he had once thought. And more surprising than that, he was learning to enjoy it. One day he faced the fact that this was serious and he was hooked. No longer was he just being nice to this crazy character, he loved me.

We met in August; we were engaged during the Kansas City Billy Graham Crusade in September, and we were married on December 15. Four months were pretty quick, but we weren't teenagers, remember. Larry's decision to marry me was not an easy one. I guess every young man at his age thinks hard about this step, but he had to face some rather unusual problems.

First, I did have an extremely strong personality. I was a performer—fairly well known—and I loved to be on the platform. Could he contend with being Karen's husband? Could he enjoy always sitting in the audience? I wanted a career, and he knew that. I told him I would never be happy knitting, cooking, and cleaning eight hours a day. He knew he wouldn't be able to take away that drive, that desire to be in front of people. Is this what he wanted?

Second, did he want a fat wife? This was the most difficult part of his decision. He already knew what it was like to be with me in a restaurant or a department store and be stared at the whole time. Did he want to live the rest of his life like that? He wondered what I really looked like, how the weight would affect our marriage, how his friends and family would react to me. And was he willing to accept the fact that I would probably always be fat? He knew that marriage in itself wouldn't make me lose weight.

As he watched from his seat, did he really want to be the husband of that 300-pound woman, decked out in a caftan and dangling earrings, standing center stage, microphone in hand, doing a comedy fat routine? What was his answer as he listened to all around him laugh at her jokes?

"I love you," he said. After all of that, he still wanted to marry me.

We have been married ten years now, and it was only as I picked Larry's thoughts to write this book that I truly realized that, after all my years of searching, he was really the first person who loved me just the way I was. Both before and after we were married I was so busy focusing on my own hang-ups that I never knew it and never appreciated it. I'm so grateful that God didn't allow me to ruin everything before I made that discovery.

Larry took me home to meet his family. What a day that was! I had never been in a small town longer than it took to drive through one. I knew very little about small-town people or their lifestyle. I did what I thought I should and dressed up for the occasion. After all, I wanted to make a good impression.

When we drove across the railroad tracks and toward the town square where we saw the banner

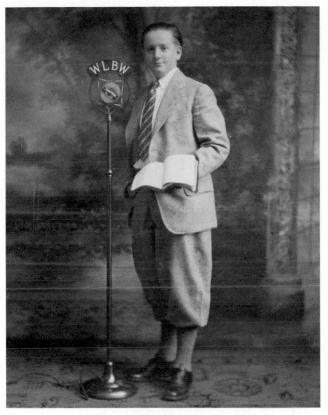

Junior Lehman—The Boy Preacher—at fifteen years of age.

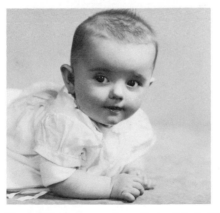

Karen Mae Lehman, born December 1, 1942.

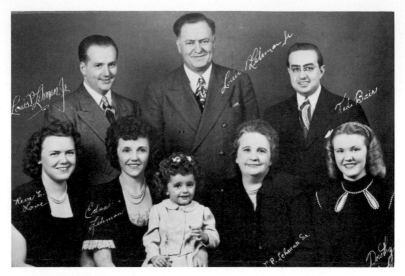

The "Bit of Heaven" radio team in 1945.

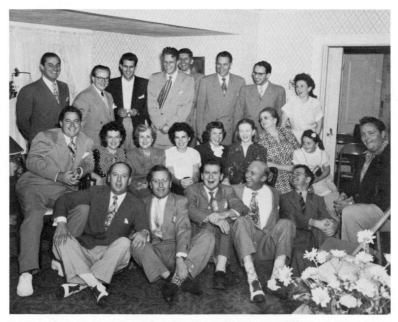

During a Billy Graham Crusade in Portland, Oregon, in 1949, our home was the scene of a social gathering for the Billy Graham team. This gathering was the kind of thing that characterized the "Christian world" I grew up in.

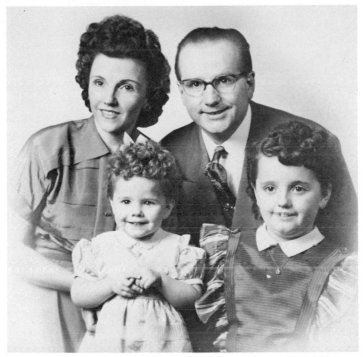

It was after our move to Grand Rapids that I began to gain weight. Here, I was nine and my sister Cheri, two.

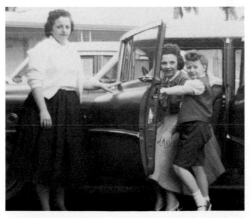

In 1957, at age fifteen, I was preparing to return to the Christian boarding school I attended for three years. Being overweight had become an inescapable fact.

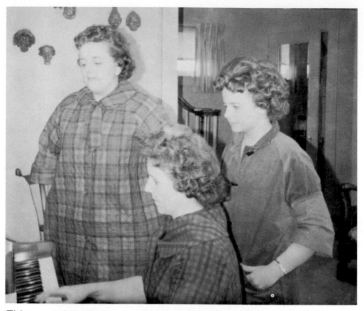

This was taken during my first year in Bible college—age eighteen.

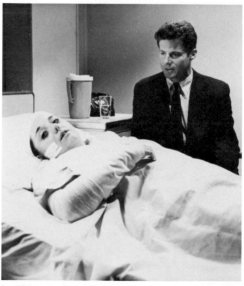

In 1964, during this scene in the film "World's Apart," I first realized God's love for a fat, mixed-up preacher's kid.

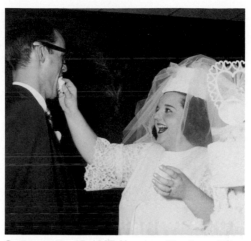

On December 15, 1967, I became Mrs. Larry Wise.

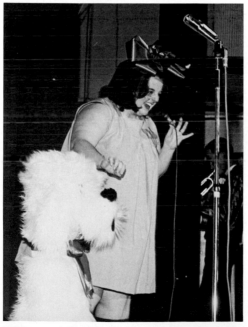

While on staff with the Kansas City Youth For Christ, I had many opportunities to refine the image I had begun to develop years earlier as the funny fat person.

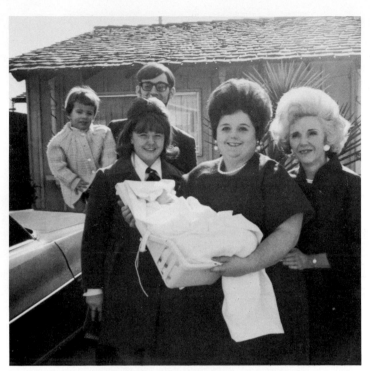

In 1970, Melissa Dee Wise was one and a half years old and her brother Jason, three months. Their mother (here with my sister Cheri and my mother on either side) was soon to weigh in at 340 pounds.

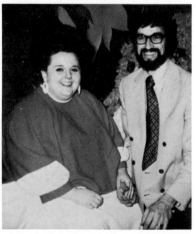

1974—340 pounds and holding.

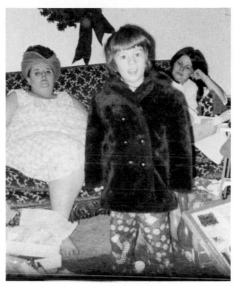

Here's what it's *really* like to be fat.

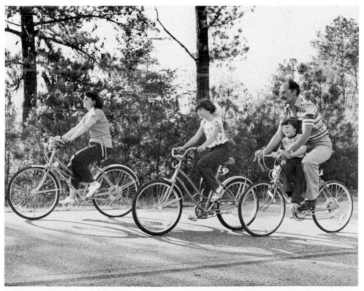

After four years of dieting, at 130 pounds, I can enjoy my family in ways I never dreamed possible.

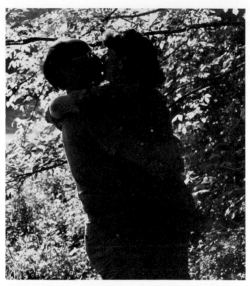

Being able to put his arms *all* the way around me and pick me up were things my husband never dreamed possible!

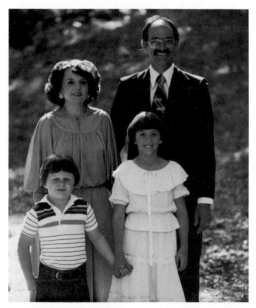

The Wise family, 1978.

telling us it was homecoming weekend, I already knew I was in foreign territory.

Larry had told his family I was heavy, but I'm sure it didn't prepare them for what they saw when we walked through the front door of his mother's house. In all my finest dingle-dangles, I waddled in to meet all the relatives who were dressed in casual attire for the homecoming parade. What a study in contrasts! Their eyes got fairly big— probably just to take it all in—but no one expressed aloud any shock, and the festivities continued. Throughout the whole day I was exposed to new and exciting events. The main attraction, of course, was a parade made up of children riding bicycles with crepe paper through the spokes, children walking their pets, and floats consisting of pick-ups with straw in the back end, which served as a platform for several costumed teenagers. There was not one helium-filled balloon! I was also escorted around the square to see the homemade quilts in the store windows, and the day was highlighted by a cup of coffee at the Cozy Cafe.

If you think I was often stared at in Kansas City, you should have been in Fredonia, Kansas, that day.

I have since come to appreciate the homemade quilts of his family and their antique furniture, but on that first day the only thing that came to mind was, "What am I getting myself into?"

Larry's family was far more concerned about my career than my weight. Being a musician and actress-type didn't sound too stable to them. I'm sure they felt it would have been much smarter for their baby brother to have married one of those other lovely, quiet, normal girls he had brought home. I had to learn to understand a different life-style, and they have found over the years that I am not a hopeless case.

Our wedding, as you might imagine, was a full-scale production. We had special lighting, a twelve-voice choir, and a brass ensemble, fully equipped with kettle drums that threatened the total audience with cardiac arrest just before I came down the aisle. I wrote all the music, and I also sang. We got married in the Youth For Christ auditorium, which required twelve ushers and microphones for all participants. My father married us and Al Metsker took part as well.

I was so well known for my tent dresses that I had my wedding dress made to follow suit and had attached to the back a long, cathedral-length lace train. There were two train bearers that held it out in back, not because that was the formal thing to do, but rather because it camouflaged my size. I also planned the ceremony so that we faced the audience the entire time. I figured if people could watch our expressions, maybe they wouldn't notice my shape.

Many of the things I will say in the rest of this chapter Larry and I never said aloud until recently. He tried not to hurt me. I kept overcompensating, and a lot of damage was done. Maybe you will benefit from our mistakes.

We spent our honeymoon in California. Even though Larry had decided to accept my weight, there are always things in any situation in life that you never really know if you can handle until you have to.

He may have tried to imagine what I looked like under the caftan or tent dress, but he wasn't prepared for it. From day one, even though he loved me and was proud of my accomplishments and abilities, he found it difficult to find me attractive as a woman. My arms were the size of most people's legs, my thighs were immense, and my stomach hung halfway to my knees. There was no shape to me. I was just a blob of flab and stretch marks, and when you took off the colorful drapings and took away the coiffured hair and the make-up, it wasn't a very pretty sight.

He really tried to make it happen at first, but this is something he never adjusted to. Obligation rather than passion was the motivation for our sexual activity.

Three months after our marriage I became pregnant. I had a normal pregnancy—no trouble with high blood pressure or swelling, which had been expected. I quit working when I was several months along and even learned to knit and enjoy some domesticity.

The day before Christmas, 1968, at 8:00 in the morning—three weeks overdue—I entered the hospital to have labor induced. After such a perfect nine months with no problems at all, no one was prepared for what happened. Everything went wrong.

I was in labor for a day and a half. The baby was literally stuck in the birth canal. I was so fat, even on the inside, that there wasn't enough room for her to get through. For awhile they thought they would lose the baby; then they thought they would lose both of us. They knew one thing for sure, if the baby made it at all, she would have a head like a cucumber and severe brain damage. They considered a Caesarian section, but the baby was down too far. My doctor tried everything. After X rays, thirty-six hours of labor, and additional examinations, they decided to give me an hour, and if nothing changed, they would operate, which certainly meant losing the baby and endangering my life as well because of her position.

I must take this opportunity to tell you what was going through my mind during those long hours. When I was telling you about my time in Houston, you will remember I told you that many times I thought that someday God would get me for what I had done. Ever since then, one of the problems I had had, even as a Christian, was in the area of forgiveness. My problem wasn't, and isn't, unique. A lot of Christians experience the same thing; that's why I mention it. When I accepted Christ as my personal Savior, I asked Him to forgive me of my sin. The Bible says that when you ask His forgiveness, He removes your sin as far as the East is from the West. It also says He remembers those sins no more. I believed that He forgave me—but remember them no more? I struggled with that. Boy, I remembered them!

There were always times when I felt God would still punish me for what I had done. I didn't deserve anything better. I thought for awhile that probably God wouldn't allow me to get married, and when I got married I immediately thought He wouldn't let me have any children, and when I got pregnant, I knew that He would probably punish me by letting the baby die.

And as I lay there hour after hour, knowing I was in trouble and knowing that the baby's life was in danger, what do you think my conclusion was? "God hasn't forgotten either. I'm going to have to pay."

Finally the hour was up and my condition hadn't changed. Everyone assumed the doctor would operate. He walked into the room, stood there for a minute and said, "We're going to wheel you to the delivery room. Nothing has really changed, but I just can't operate. Somehow we're going to deliver this baby."

They told Larry not to expect anything. They had prepared him for the worst, and no one really thought there was much left of that baby.

The last thing I remember seeing were nurses lined up on either side of me, a doctor at my head, and my obstetrician at the foot of the table. And as I went under, I heard, "One, two, three, push." Later I was told they did this for fifty-five minutes.

When I came to for just a moment, there was no one left in that delivery room but my doctor and me. He simply told me I had had a baby girl, and I didn't ask any questions. I really didn't want to know her condition.

At 4:30 the next morning they started to wheel me back to my room. On the way, I decided I wanted to know how bad the outcome was, and so

I asked the nurses if they could take me by the nursery so I could see my baby. I expected them to put me off until morning so that I could rest before getting the bad news, but instead they turned the bed in the direction of the crying babies.

I was lying there waiting, preparing myself for anything, when they held this beautiful baby up in front of me. Her head was as round as a rubber ball. There was not a scratch, a bruise, or a mark on her anywhere. Her dark brown eyes were wide open and she was moving all four perfect arms and legs at the same time. I was overwhelmed and started to cry. One of the nurses looked at me and said, "I hope you realize, young lady, that nobody in this hospital has an explanation for this strong, healthy baby."

I did.

She was a symbol of God's total forgiveness. How God loved me! Melissa Dee Wise, seven pounds, eleven ounces, was born at 11:50 P.M. on Christmas Day, 1968.

I was told not to have any more children, and so we didn't wait long to start adoption proceedings. When Melissa was a year and a half, we got a call that our little boy was waiting for us to pick him up.

He was only forty-eight hours old when we got him. His body didn't fit his skin yet; he was completely bald and was so tiny I thought he would break. We named him Jason Garth.

At 8 and 10, both children continue to be talented and intelligent today, an objective opinion, of course.

These ten years of marriage and motherhood

have been filled with ups and downs—in fact, a lot of downs. You will be shocked to know that my husband isn't perfect, and some of our problems have been his. But a lot of them have been mine, and a lot of mine have been because of my weight. Being fat affected my total relationship with my husband and my children.

I came into this marriage with security only in a platform image. Because I was fat so long before I married, I didn't see much worth in me as a real person. In my eyes I was a failure. I didn't like myself at all. I didn't know how to really love. I didn't know how to accept love. I couldn't believe that anybody *could* really love me; therefore, I couldn't accept it. And, likewise, I didn't feel that anybody could want what I had to give.

It was impossible to believe that Larry wanted to be seen with me. And whether he said so or not, I knew my weight bothered and embarrassed him. There is nothing in a marriage relationship that is not affected by an attitude like that.

I was also suffering from the results of that protective shield I had built around me some years ago. I didn't want to be hurt or rejected. I subsconsciously kept myself from giving myself totally to anyone else. I was scared to get involved even in my marriage.

And it affected the children as well. When I would go to nursery school to pick them up, the other children would gather around and make remarks like:

"Your mommy's fat."

"Your mommy dresses funny."

"Your mommy is the biggest person I have ever seen."

We would go to the grocery store, and while we were waiting in line often another child would say at the top of his voice, "Look, mommy, look at that fat lady."

Melissa would always feel bad that someone had made fun of her mother, and she would tell me she loved me even though I was fat. Larry would often have to remind the children that their mother might be heavy, but other mothers couldn't sing and play the piano.

When they started school, I avoided going to open houses and special programs so I wouldn't embarrass them. And when I was home I never went outside the door. I was missing out on whole parts of life. There were so many things Larry and I couldn't do. Our friends would include us in only the activities they knew I could handle.

The four of us never played ball or went swimming together. Just about every outdoor activity was avoided, not just because of my size but also because of the clothes I had to wear.

But the psychological problems were the ones that affected us all the most. As an adult, I still couldn't make friends, had trouble talking to any stranger on a one-to-one basis, and came home from everywhere mad because I had talked too much. I was uncomfortable in any situation I didn't control.

I was always trying to overcompensate or prove something, even with my own family. And I was defensive. No one could criticze me for anything. I would fall apart, and then attack the other person. No wonder my husband didn't communicate.

We had good days, good friends, and good times, but our marriage was very rocky. We have been on the very brink of divorce twice and talked about it several other times. During all these years I did a lot of speaking, giving my testimony, singing, and doing fashion shows for overweight women.

My testimonies were not insincere. God had done a lot for me. I was not playing a game, and I know the Lord has used me over the years. But I didn't let Him do for me all He wanted to do. I had always been so critical of all those people who got on platforms and preached certain things and still had holes in their lives. I'm not condoning any of them or myself, but I sure do understand what its like to be there. I felt like a hypocrite. I sometimes wondered why someone didn't laugh out loud when I stood in front of a group of people at 340 pounds and said, "Whatever your problem is, God can solve it." Sure it bothered me. It also bothered me that even though I could tell my story up to a certain point, I had nothing to say about what God had done with my marriage.

I started to feel differently about my childhood idols whom I had felt let me down. I know one thing for sure, if you're waiting for the perfect preacher, speaker, or gospel singer to come along before you decide whether there is any truth in what God can do, you'll wait forever.

God is still working on all of us. Four years ago I had a lot to share about what God had done for me. Four years later and 210 pounds lighter, I still have a lot to share. That's where the genuine stuff is at. Can you tell that God is working?

During this period in my life, I was aware more than ever how my own family was affected by all of the things I still struggled with, and every night I would pray and ask God to help me conquer some of those things the next day. But I wasn't ready yet to face the fact that until I let God do something about the weight, I would never get rid of all the side effects.

CHAPTER 8

SQUEEZING
MY WAY THROUGH

Fat people have a unique problem. First, they have a problem that everybody knows they could do something about, "if they really wanted to." Second, they can never hide it—never, never ever!

The alcoholic can be sober for a few hours and the people around him for that period of time may never know he drinks. The lady with a bad case of nerves can at times get herself together enough to pull the wool over the eyes of her dinner guests

The fat person never has that privilege.

Twenty-four hours a day, wherever you go, you are a walking billboard continually announcing to the world:

"I am a person who has a problem I cannot control."

You know it, I know it, and, more importantly, I know that you know it. Live with that for twenty-six years and see if it doesn't affect your mind. And live with all the logistical problems of being 5 feet

4 inches tall and weighing 340 pounds and see if it doesn't affect your life-style.

I very seldom sat in chairs with arms; some I couldn't get into at all. If I did manage to sit in one, after a few minutes I would be in pain and the arms would leave marks in the sides of my thighs. When I would try to get up I had to pry myself out or take the chair with me. Aluminum lawn chairs with the little woven seats had to be avoided altogether, and getting on a bar stool was a comedy routine all in itself. If I ever got up on one, the stool completely disappeared.

I backed into restrooms on the airplane, because once the door was closed, I couldn't turn around. I always had to have a seat-belt extension when I flew, and I couldn't use lap trays on airplanes because my stomach was in the way. If I was on a long flight, I would have to get up and walk around every hour because my legs would go numb from the pressure of the arms of the seats. Sometimes I would get bruises from the buttons and stereo adjustments on the inside of those arms.

I couldn't get into booths in restaurants and could only drive certain cars. Getting in and out of the backseat of a two-door car was like something out of a slap-stick comedy routine, and once wedged into a bathtub it was impossible to move around.

Revolving doors and the little revolving entrance gates in airports, drug stores, and amusement parks were sometimes impossible and many times difficult and painful. I simply avoided them.

I couldn't wear shoes with buckles or walk very

far without my feet hurting, and I huffed and
puffed from just putting on my nylons.

Just sitting in any feminine manner was a chore.
To keep my knees together on a platform or in a
crowded room hurt so much that it many times
ruined a whole evening.

I always checked for wobbly piano benches,
frail-looking chairs, and beds with weak slats. I
had to completely avoid boats, amusement rides,
picnic tables, and school desks. I always tried to sit
in an aisle seat wherever I went.

I wouldn't walk to a front seat of any meeting
unless I was on the program. I tried not to walk
across a room in front of people. I never introduced myself to anyone and never attended any
function simply as a participant unless I went with
someone I knew.

Not many people ever knew these things. In
fact, most people—even my close friends—
thought my weight didn't present much of a problem for me. Even when things were logistically
difficult or even painful, I carried it off so that no
one knew it.

I will say that I always had a lot of energy—pure
sugar energy, I'm sure—and my life was usually
busier than most other people's. But I was out of
breath and uncomfortable most of the time. After a
number of years of living like this, I learned to
avoid a chair or a middle-of-the-row seat without
anyone knowing what I had done. If I couldn't, I
always had a joke to carry me through.

The things I couldn't participate in anyway—
such as sports—were to those around me simply

things in which I wasn't interested. It was much
easier to build an image that put down these things
than to say I wanted to participate but couldn't.

I became an expert at overcompensation. Never
could I walk into a room or meet someone new and
simply ride on what I looked like. I had to prove
that even though I looked bad, I was worth something. My personality as a result was loud, overbearing, pushy, opinionated, overwhelming, and
dominating. Fun at parties, but a little hard to take
on an everyday basis.

I now wore nothing but caftans, which in my
condition was better than slacks, believe me. The
caftans were colorful and always hung below
dangling earrings and a hairdo piled high on my
head in a mild attempt at offsetting the width.

Here are a few of the remarks I heard so often:

"You carry your weight so well, and it doesn't seem
to bother you,"

or

"You dress so well. Even though you're heavy,
you're always well groomed,"

or

"I've never met anyone as big as you with so much
ambition; you're a successful person. You've accomplished a lot for your age,"

or

"I guess you're proof that there are fat people who
aren't bothered by their weight,"

or the winner

"You have such a pretty face."

All these comments proved I had worked very

hard on my overcompensation, and most of the time it worked very well for me. But the overcompensation wasn't me—it was an image.

Let me tell you about the person that lived under the caftan. Let me tell you about the miserable Karen. Let me tell you what it's *really* like to be fat.

It's being tired of overcompensating and wanting so desperately just to be accepted for what you are.

It's not being able to accept *yourself* for what you are.

It's wanting to be loved as a woman, but not being able to accept that love because you can't believe anybody would love you.

It's being stared at all the time; and having children point you out (loudly) to their mothers in the grocery store.

It's learning to joke about your body to put other people at ease.

It's walking around with cuts on the insides of your legs from girdles and nylons and never having those cuts heal because they break open every time you walk.

It's being asked to entertain at a party, but never being asked to join two or three ladies for lunch at the country club.

It's buying clothes only where they sell big-girl sizes and underwear to match.

It's wanting to know your husband is proud to be with you and knowing that isn't possible.

It's wanting to get up out of a chair gracefully.

It's wanting to participate in a world you've only

watched—a world of people who swim, ride bikes with their kids, and go for long walks in the park.

It's wanting to bend over to dust the bottom rung of a chair without getting out of breath.

It's wanting your kids to be able to sit on your lap comfortably.

It's wanting desperately to be in a crowded room and be one of the crowd.

And most of all it's wanting to feel like something other than a failure. It's wanting to be able to look in the mirror and say, "I like you, Karen. I don't hate you anymore."

The one thing fat people have in common is that they hate themselves. They hate themselves because they're a failure. They've proven over and over to themselves that when it comes to licking that problem, they can do nothing but fail. And at thirty-one years old that's where I was: 340 pounds and a failure as a person, as a mother, as a wife, as a friend. Nothing I had accomplished in my life added up to anything, because I knew that the one thing that affected my whole life—the thing that had hold of my mind and was slowly killing my body—I had no control over. What else was that but total failure?

Then, one day I heard they were performing an operation called an intestinal bypass on people like me. I was convinced that this was my last hope and looked into it right away. I found a doctor, passed the tests, and put my life on the line willingly for what I thought was the answer. Just the anticipation changed my mental attitude. Why, this was a dream come true. I could have the operation, eventually be the person I wanted to be, and still eat hot-fudge sundaes, cheesecake, and baked potatoes with sour cream and butter. I was ecstatic about this new way of losing weight, which wouldn't require my developing any self-discipline, or making any changes in my life-style.

All the stories about people being sick for long periods of time didn't phase me in the least. I didn't care about that as long as I would eventually be thin.

The surgery was performed. All went well. I recovered quickly, was sent home, and was on cloud nine as I watched the pounds begin to come off. I was like a new person, convinced that my life-long dream was at last coming true. Someday I would be beautiful.

I shed thirty to forty pounds with ease and then, suddenly, everything stopped. I didn't lose another pound. Everything stabilized and quit. I had read that sometimes the operation didn't work, but that could never happen to me—not me, Lord, please not me.

But, it did happen to me, and I still weighed 300 pounds. The period of depression that followed is very hard to put into words. My last hope was gone. I was fat, ugly, and unlovable even in God's eyes.

More than anything, I knew that I didn't want to live the rest of my life in that condition. I also knew that I didn't have what it would take to lose 225 pounds.

What was I to do, kill myself? It didn't sound bad. In fact, that sounded a lot easier than losing weight.

At this point, desperately, I cried to God.

"Show me something, anything in myself worth fighting for.

"Tell me Lord what to do. I don't know what to do.

"I can't live like this. Please help me. I don't want to be fat.

"Is there anything You can do for me?"

I wish I could tell you that I said "Amen" and everything was different. I wish I could tell you a flash of lightning hit and took away my appetite.

But none of that happened.

Yes, God performed a miracle, a slow but real one.

The first part of the miracle was painful. God helped me face reality.

CHAPTER 9

REALITY IS PAINFUL

The pain of seeing yourself as you really are is deep and cutting. I shed many tears, and I hurt from humiliation. The guilt I experienced when I felt I had thrown my life away was heavier than all the other guilt I had carried.

But God graciously helped me stare two important facts in the face and deal with them. Only then could He begin to heal the damage, take away the hurt, and show me His unlimited forgiveness. First, I had to be aware of exactly how bad my problem was and how severely it was affecting my life. My weight made every decision in life for me.

It told me where I could go and where I couldn't go.

It told me what chair I could sit in and what chair I couldn't sit in.

It dictated what kind of car I could drive, what job I could have, what activities I could participate in, what friends I could have, what I could do for my children, and what kind of wife I could be.

There wasn't one area of my life that was not affected by my problem. I had been willing to accept second best in everything in order to eat.

I had exchanged my birthright of being thin and normal for the pottage of a bag of chocolate-covered peanuts. I was a foodaholic. Food had precisely as much control over me as drugs have over an addict. It had totally drained my worth as a person. My life was controlled by what I ate and by the fact I couldn't quit.

First, I had to admit I loved food more than my husband and my children. If I didn't I would have lost the weight in order to make their lives better and happier.

I let *my* weight control *their* lives, at least to a certain extent. They did what I could do and went where I could go.

Second, I had to stop blaming everyone else for my problems.

I was thirty-one years old. My mother didn't gain my weight; my schoolteacher didn't gain it; my father didn't gain it; my husband didn't gain it—I gained it. I put on every pound all by myself. Me—just me—and it was my fault and not anyone else's.

It was time to quit excusing myself for not being what I ought to be, just because I could make a list of others who weren't what they ought to be.

I've known a lot of people who have gone to psychiatrists for help with their weight problem. Most of them come out with twenty reasons why they are fat and no answer as to what to do about it. Some people have found out they are fat because their grandma was a good cook or because they read Little Lulu comic strips when they were young. Others are fat because they were reminded too often of the starving Chinese children, or they churned too much butter on the farm. I'm sure if you looked hard enough you would find someone who is fat because they sat next to a fat person in church.

Sure, there were many things in my life that could have contributed to my problem, and I could have listed them accurately. But *I* still weighed 300 pounds.

And knowing *why* I was fat didn't make it go away.

It was also time for me to quit playing the role of a frustrated actress. The Christian world hadn't stopped me from getting a college degree. My parents had never told me I couldn't study directing. No one had ever prohibited me from becoming a good writer instead of a mediocre one. It had always been easier to find excuses than to work hard. It had always been less difficult to develop self-pity than self-discipline, and it had always been safer to hide and eat than to compete and fail.

My father told me when I was thirteen years old that for every ounce of talent there must be an ounce of self-discipline. When he told me that, I thought he was crazy.

And at thirty-one, in addition to being fat, I also faced the fact that I had always slid by, doing some things well and nothing skillfully because I had taken the talent God had given me and only played with it.

There comes a time with any problem when you simply can't pass the buck any longer. As an adult you have to accept the problem as yours and ask

God to help you become the person you know He wants you to be in spite of all the odds.

If God isn't strong enough to win out over all you have been, all the disappointments you have lived through, all the weaknesses you still have, then He really isn't what you say He is. This realization brought me to a turning point.

I had been "hypocrite hunting" all my life. As a preacher's kid, I had spent hours of time down through the years pointing out all the people who didn't live what they preached. I had worked so hard at not being one of them that I had surpassed them and left them in the dust.

Oh, I didn't want to face that—it was so hard. I cried, and I avoided it. I tried to come up with a better explanation, one that would make me look better, but finally I had to hit it head on.

"God is capable of handling anything," I said to groups of people. God is capable of handling anything *but my weight problem,* I would say to myself.

Did I believe God could handle the impossible or didn't I? If I didn't, there wasn't much truth in what I said I believed. If I did believe it, then it was time to let Him work on me—for my benefit, not for anyone else's.

I didn't want to be thin for my mother or my husband or my children as much as I wanted to be thin for *me.* I needed that healing. I needed a new life and a new attitude. And most of all, for my own faith and spiritual growth, I needed to know that God doesn't just work miracles in the lives of other people, but that He was able to work a miracle in me.

I decided to see if it would really work. For the first time in my life I was willing to believe that God could give me what I needed to lick this problem. The thought of losing 225 pounds blew my mind, but somehow God was already changing my attitude.

I have never asked God to take my appetite away. My first prayer was for God to tip the scales by changing my priorities. Food had been most important; what God wanted me to be had been second. I wanted the first things reversed.

And that was my request of God. Change the priorities.

CHAPTER 10

WE'RE GOING
TO MAKE IT THIS TIME

And so the dieting began.

We also moved from Kansas City to Atlanta at about the same time. My marriage was at about the lowest ebb it had ever been. The three or four months preceding the move were horrible. In fact, I contemplated not moving and going my separate way. At the time, I didn't know why we stayed together, but I knew I couldn't leave.

We were also in the middle of a difficult financial crisis. I tell you this because most people keep waiting until the perfect time to lose weight, a time when there is no emotional pressure, nothing tearing them apart. But not so with me. If I would have waited, I would probably be back up to 340 pounds.

And that, too, is part of the miracle, for in the middle of eight good reasons why I couldn't, I started to diet successfully.

The first thing I had to do was get off of sugar. I had saturated my body with it for twenty-six years. I actually went through a withdrawal period. I was nauseous, tired, and very emotional. Day by day

God helped me through it until my body started to acclimate.

I also cut out bread and potatoes. For me to walk hand in hand every day with just meat, vegetables, and salads was as unnatural as Dolly Parton and Leonard Bernstein performing together. It was by far the hardest thing I had ever done.

The normal evangelical prescription of prayer in the morning and again at bedtime was not sufficient for me. I was too weak. This is when I began using what I call "on-the-spot" praying. Every time I sat down at the table, alone or with others, I would pray my way through. The people sitting beside me never knew it, but I asked God for help constantly.

> "Dear Lord, keep my hands on my lap. Don't let me reach for that roll."

> "Dear Lord, help me to order what I should; help me not to order dessert even though everyone else is."

> "Dear Lord, help me not to clean my plate."

> "Help me remember my goal, what I want to be."

And if you think I had to pray when I was in a crowd, that was nothing compared to how I had to pray when I was alone. Alone is always worse. It's just you, God, and all those fat rationalizations. I caught myself saying, "No one will ever know if I eat just this one piece of pie, these two small pieces of candy, just three tablespoons of ice cream." I would stand with my hand on the refrigerator door and pray, "God, don't let me open it." I would look at a bowl of ice cream already dished up and pray, "Don't let me eat it," and found I had the strength to put it back.

Through the suggestion of John Haggai—a man whom I greatly respect and whom I work for but also consider a great friend—I also began to learn about verbal affirmations. For so many years I had told myself the only thing I could do was fail, that now I had to begin to convince myself that I could win.

The reprogramming began, undoing twenty-six years of self-degradation. Every morning I started by looking at myself in the mirror and saying, "Karen, you're going to make it this time." When I wanted to eat I would remind myself, "Karen, you have what it takes. You're going to make it this time." I don't even know how much *I* believed it at first; it seemed like such a large task. But God believed in me and never took His hand off me.

When you weigh 300 pounds, no one notices if you've lost ten, and it was a long time before the changes were evident to anyone but me. These were long, lonely days. I wanted people to notice how well I was doing, but my caftans still hid everything well, even the improvements. Also, you have to remember that even after I had lost 100 pounds, to people I had never met before I was still a fat person.

And I must admit that there were days when the "on-the-spot" praying and the verbal affirmations didn't work because they weren't sincere, days when I just wanted to eat. There were those days when I would feel sorry for myself, days when I felt no one cared if I lost anyway, days when I got sick and tired of being on a diet.

There were times when I let myself enjoy being a martyr, using the old line that "no one understands me" nor my problems nor how hard it is to stick with a diet. When I felt like that, I didn't pray or talk to myself. I simply didn't want any help; I only wanted to eat. And what a binge I would go on. I would eat everything in sight. But I would get sick quicker than I once had and would soon be disgusted with myself.

After about the second binge, however, I recognized a change in me, a *real* change, and how excited I was! Always before when I tried to diet, the first binge was always the end. It was always a sign that I had failed again, and so I would quit. Now I found myself thinking logically. I had lost twenty pounds. The most I could have gained on my binge was two or three pounds. I was still seventeen pounds ahead. All I had to do was get up the next morning and start again—and I did! I wanted to shout, "Look everybody. Look what's happening to me. God has given me the ability to stick with it even when I fall on my face." But I didn't shout it; I didn't figure anyone else would think it was such a big deal. But it was to me.

God was answering my prayers. He was beginning to change me. I was worth something. God thought so, anyway.

I have to mention the helpful and unhelpful

people I encountered on my way down to 130 pounds. Ironically, a lot of the unhelpful ones were the people who were always after me to lose. Of all things, they would coax me to eat!

There is one example that stands out above many others. One friend, who when I was my heaviest, always brought up the subject of how pretty I could be if I would just take off the pounds. After I had lost about fifty of those pounds, my husband and I were at her home for dinner. When it was time for dessert I declined, which I was learning to do. Well, she started in with the usual "a little piece won't hurt you" stuff, and when I still declined, she really zeroed in.

"I spent all afternoon on this. It's a new recipe. I will really feel hurt if you don't taste it." I reminded her that she was the one who was always after me to lose, and I asked her to forgive me, but told her I wouldn't eat any. Instead of being proud of me, she actually became very cool. It is said that people don't like to drink alone, but apparently people don't like to eat desserts alone, either!

Most folks are uncomfortable eating dessert in front of someone who has passed it up. They always say they feel bad eating in front of the dieter, but the truth usually is that they feel bad about eating it themselves. If they can get you to cheat, they feel a lot better.

And then there are those women who have encouraged you to lose, but when you get too close to their weight category, they start telling you not to lose anymore. Even if you are still overweight, they will say you look terrific and that you will look bad if you get any thinner. After all, they have always looked better than you, and they don't want it to end up the other way around!

Then, there are always those few who feel it's a shame that you are losing your image. They try to convince you they liked you fat, that the old you was the real Karen. And the one question I have answered over and over again is, "Do you think your personality will change? Do you think you'll lose your sense of humor?" (Stay tuned, I'll answer those questions in the next chapter.)

But then there were all those helpful people along the way, those who noticed when I lost another pound or two or when I had a new dress a size smaller. They were lifesavers. When I wanted to give up, many times it was just a word of encouragement that helped me over the hump.

On one of those hungry days, I stepped into the elevator in the building where I worked, and the man who rode up with me looked at me and said, "You're looking terrific, prettier every day." That's all it took.

Other friends learned to eat while I drank a cup of coffee, and they didn't make a major production over it, which I appreciated. My husband started going to the ice cream store and coming out with three cones, instead of four, without any discussion.

I guess I would say that the people who were most helpful were those who knew when to fuss over me and when not to. Most people didn't realize that in dealing with a dieter it takes the helpful combination of encouragement and keeping your mouth shut.

I also became very thankful for my job. One of the best ways to stay away from food is to stay busy and not to sit and look at it all day.

I did not use diet pills of any kind, and I don't recommend them to anyone. I did take them at various times in my life, but they sent me higher than a kite and I became immune to them after several weeks. A lot of people I know have gotten hooked on the energy kick they give and have suffered deep depression when they have quit taking them.

I lost slowly but consistently—a pound or two a week. This is probably why my face, at least, doesn't sag. (I'll talk about the rest of me a bit later.)

Month after month went by. The cravings got less severe and the binges farther and farther apart. And finally I really began to look different. When I got into a size 18 dress, I decided the caftans had to go. In addition to that, I could now wear panty hose—the eighth wonder of the world.

I bought the first street-length dress I had worn since before my six and one-half year old boy was born. Standing in my bedroom, I felt awkward and half naked. I didn't know whether or not to go outside dressed like that. But I was proud and full of anticipation. I walked out the front door and walked to the car, and my little boy looked at me very strangely and said, "Mommy, your legs are showing." He was right, but no one laughed at me the whole day. No one looked at me like I wasn't dressed right. In fact, I felt kind of normal, like a regular person.

Do you have any idea what an experience that was? Sure, I was still overweight, but I wasn't a freak any longer. I *was* going to make it this time.

The last year has brought about the drastic changes. I couldn't get rid of those thirty-eight caftans fast enough. I have gone from that size 18 to a 9 Junior. My shoes are two sizes smaller, and my legs show almost all the time!

People have noticed the change and have told me so. My children have been proud to introduce their mother to their schoolteachers. My husband has a wife who doesn't get stared at, and I have reached the place where I can eat basically one meal a day at noon and take vitamin and protein supplements without getting hungry.

But best of all, Karen is a person she likes.

And even now I practice that on-the-spot praying. There are times when I wish I could eat like other people; there are days when I would like a hot fudge sundae. But I wouldn't trade what God has helped me become for all the chocolate in Hershey, Pennsylvania.

About six months ago I was driving down one of the junk-food highways during my lunch hour. I decided I had done so well and had stuck with my diet so long that I figured one chocolate malt wouldn't hurt. If I didn't eat supper it wouldn't put a pound on me. So I pulled my car into a long line of others waiting for service at a drive-up window at a hamburger stand. I waited and waited, all the time knowing I was doing something stupid. When I was almost to the window, I said to myself, "You've come so far, you're not going to blow it now, are you?"

"Even if this doesn't put a pound on you, it will get the sugar running in your system again. God, don't let me be so dumb."

With that, I pulled my car out of line and drove away.

I went instead to a small coffee shop across the street for a cup of coffee. When I walked in, I didn't see a soul. I was the only customer, and there was no waitress in sight. I sat down in an end booth, and almost immediately a woman about my age came out of the back room. She weighed approximately 325 pounds. She was dressed in a pair of slacks and a knit top that didn't meet in the middle, and her apron strings were pinned together in the back. I could count every roll of fat as she shuffled toward me. She slowly got me my cup of coffee and decided since I was the only one in there she would tell me her problems.

As I sat there, I listened to her tell me how tired she was, how she lived with her mother, and how her whole routine consisted of cooking, sleeping, and eating. She had never seen me before, and she ended her conversation by saying, "My mother keeps telling me to lose weight, but I tell her she doesn't understand. And I don't suppose you do either, lady, as pretty as you are."

As she turned away, my eyes filled with tears and I thanked the Lord for helping me to drive across the street. I also thanked Him for how far

He had brought me. And I also asked Him to never let me forget what it had been like to be fat, both for my benefit and for the benefit of all those I would meet in the days and months ahead who feel no one understands.

CHAPTER 11

MY NEW LIFE

A few months ago I was invited to Florida to speak to a group of people on the subject of weight loss. That even sounds strange to write it. These people didn't want me to sing or tell my life story or be funny. They just wanted me to tell people why and how I had lost so many pounds.

I have stood in front of people many times in my life, but as I sat on the front row waiting to be introduced, I felt more nervous than I had felt in years. I was able to keep my emotions under control only until I actually started to speak. I'm afraid I'll have to admit, I just stood there and cried. I looked out over those three hundred people and it suddenly hit me that they had all come to hear Karen Wise speak on weight loss.

In all of the dreams I had had in my life, I had never dreamed of this. Many years before I had given up dreaming of ever losing weight at all. And now here I was, standing there in a size 10 dress, with my hair casually blown dry instead of piled on my head, tears streaming down my face, telling people what it was like to be fat and how wonderful it is to be thin. I suppose this was the ultimate experience of my long haul and of this last year of great transition.

Let me remind you that even though I have been losing for about three and a half years, it has just been in the last twelve to fifteen months that the real changes in my life-style and thought patterns have taken place. Until I got down to about a size 16 dress, I still was a very fat person in my mind. I knew I was going to make it, but I didn't face all the mental adjustments until I really began to look and feel like other people.

This last year has been filled with many discoveries about the real me that got covered up by image and overcompensating. It has been filled with a lot of mental reprogramming, fun experiences, and many, many miles of progress. I have also been able to ask God for some help I've never asked for before and have had to go to Him to see me through some feelings and insecurities I've never experienced before. Most of all, I've thanked Him a lot.

A little over a year ago, I was performing at a Christian supper club for three nights a week doing an hour and a half of music and my fat routine. Even though I was losing weight, I was still heavy enough to continue doing this routine even while I was dieting. People who knew I was dieting and who were noticing the drastic changes began asking, "What are you going to do when you have to give this up? What are you going to do when you can't be funny any more?" I really didn't know. I guess that's why I kept doing it.

As I was rehearsing my routine I began to find

that I was having to work at appearing funny and fat and awkward. In fact, I wore caftans in order to look bigger. In my routine I usually sat on a bar stool, which had always been difficult for me to get on and off of, but now I had to make it *look* difficult. I had a song, too, that I had written and used for years as the opening to my routine:

> Why should I be thin when I can be fat and beautiful,
> When I walk in the room, people stare
> Why should I be thin when I can be fat and beautiful,
> To me a Miss America's a spare.
> Why should I create a shape that dazzles people here and there
> When I worked so hard on one that dazzles all
> Oh, why should I run a mile and ruin a perfect style
> Just to look like every other girl.
>
> *Chorus:*
> Well, I'm not going to do it
> I'm not going to do it
> I'm going to stand my ground pound by pound
> And be the biggest, most beautiful girl in the world.

Now when I sang it from the piano, I was having to purposely sit a certain way on the bench so as to look like I covered all the territory. The lines of the routine became harder to deliver; the laughs were harder to get. By now, even though I still had a long way to go, I wasn't the biggest person in the room. Now I was beginning to see that there were people in the audience my size or bigger, and they

weren't laughing. I was thrilled with my weight
loss, but I was scared to give up the security of my
image. After all, what if I didn't have much going
for me as a regular person?

But finally I was sick of it, and I knew it was time
I found out if I could stand on my own two feet
without my crutch. One night at the end of my
third performance, after all the music and laughter
was over, I stepped back out on the platform and
made one of the most exciting announcements I
have ever made.

"You have been a special audience. You are the
last crowd that will ever see the routine I just
delivered. It's not just because I've lost a lot of
weight and it's not funny any more. As of tonight, I
am putting it away. I will never perform it again.
That is part of another era of my life. I'm walking
away from it and starting a new one. I don't want to
be fat anymore." I can't tell you what that did for
me. It was like finally saying to myself, "You're not
only going to make it, but you're going to become a
real person."

Let me insert something that happened just
three days ago. A lady called and told me she had
seen me sing and do comedy about two years ago
at a luncheon. She said she was now in charge of
finding entertainment for her church banquet, and
she wanted to know if I would come and do the
same program for them on a particular date. I told
her I wasn't doing that same program any longer
and she asked me why. I told her I had lost over
two hundred pounds and was no longer fat and
that, therefore, the old program had gone by the

wayside. After a long pause she said, "What a shame. You were so funny. You would have been just perfect for our banquet," and hung up. I was so glad I didn't fit her bill.

I'm finding that my new life presents all sorts of new experiences, and I'm not finished enjoying the excitement of them. Do you have any idea how much fun it is for me just to be able to cross my legs? I couldn't do that for seventeen years. I know it's a little thing, but I feel about that one thing like some people might feel about a new house or a new car.

I got on an airplane not long ago and I was thrilled all over again to be able to find my seat, sit down, fasten the seat belt, and just sit there—unnoticed—as the others filed by to find their places.

I have room to spare in the chairs I sit in, and more importantly I'm comfortable in them. I slide in and out from behind the steering wheel of my car without any effort. I get on a crowded elevator without having to crack a joke, and I wear shoes with three-inch heels and buckles.

Buying clothes is just plain fun. I love it. I giggle to myself when I walk into a dress department and go immediately to the rack with nine's and ten's. To be able to wear what's in style is a real privilege. I remember the day I finally got up enough nerve to walk into a store that carried junior sizes only. I had a ball, while checking from time to time to see if anybody was watching me or laughing. They weren't, of course. I bought a dress and walked out of there carrying that bag that said

"Junior Shop" on the outside so everyone could see it. I felt like a million dollars.

Finally getting my hair cut and restyled was a real boost. I discovered I didn't have to have three inches of height on top of my head anymore. I had worn curlers in my hair every night since I was about thirteen. All of a sudden I didn't have to. Needless to say, my husband didn't mind this transitional step.

I can't explain to you what it's like for me to go anywhere I want to go without being stared at or pointed at or talked about. It's overwhelming.

One night several months ago, supper was ready and I went out to find Melissa who was riding her bike. When I found her a couple of blocks up the street, I asked her to get off her bike and let me ride it. She looked at me so funny and said, "I didn't know you knew how to ride a bike." I told her that when I was a little girl I, too, had had a bike and that I was going to buy one so I could get some exercise to help take care of my thigh problem. She stood there in the middle of the street and her eyes filled up with tears, and she said, "You mean you and I will be able to do something outside together? You know we've never done anything outside together."

My weight loss has had a significant impact on my children. (Everyone knows about me: the teachers at school, their friends, the babysitter, the Sunday school teachers.) They're kind of proud of their new mommy.

When I comfortably attended the last PTA open house, I was informed I was the prettiest mommy there. I now have a pair of blue jeans, which in my children's eyes is the ultimate achievement, and I get introduced to their friends unashamedly. I still can't jump into a swimming pool with them until I have some surgery done on my legs, but I soon will.

Something most people don't think about when they see a fat person is the real damage that is done to the body by being fat for a long time. First of all, you don't weigh 340 pounds, lose it, and come out with a sixteen-year-old body. After losing weight, the skin from my stomach *still* hung down to my thighs. I had to have it surgically removed. They cut from one hip to the other and took off all the excess skin. I had a flat stomach for the first time in years. When I had been home from the hospital a few days, I noticed that the skin around the incision was beginning to turn black, and I went back in to have the doctor look at it. My skin had been stretched for so long, and it was so unhealthy, that it didn't have enough life left in it to heal properly.

I had to go back in again and they did the same thing all over, cutting back further and working with what proved to be better skin. It is still a shock to look at myself in the mirror and not see a hanging stomach. Now I look forward to having the same thing done to my thighs where there are actually handfuls of excess skin that will never tighten up. That, folks, is one of the glamorous stories about being fat.

The first question I am always asked these days is, "What does your husband think about all this?"

Just as my weight affected him and his life-style dramatically, the adjustments to the weight loss have been his as well. He is actually married to another person now, not to the one he married. There have been some fun adjustments and some not-so-fun ones.

He is proud of me, enjoys being seen with me, and is delighting in the fact that we can go places and do things we haven't been able to do before. I can now put on a pair of slacks and a sweat shirt and go bowling with him or spend a casual weekend in the mountains. He likes the clothes I'm wearing, the new hairstyle and, most of all, the new relaxed personality. He tells me I'm not as pushy or as dominating or as loud and demanding as I once was. I'm learning how to become a conversationalist instead of a performer all the time. I can lie on the couch with him, believe it or not, a pleasure we obviously had not attempted before.

It's surprising how much more room there is on his half of the bed, which used to be his quarter of the bed, and he keeps coming home to a wife wearing his shirts, which is a novelty. When he puts his arms around me, he actually puts his arms around me. He can pick me up, set me in his lap, and still breathe. And to sit next to him in the front seat I actually have to move over!

But it hasn't all been fun. I went through a couple of months when I wondered if I could compete with other women now for the attention of other men. As I was growing up, the thin ones always won out, always got the fellows I wanted. I found myself wanting to make up for that. "If I were not married," I would think to myself, "could I date anyone I wanted to?"

Men were beginning to treat me differently. I found I couldn't joke around like I had before. This is where God really had to intervene. I had never been faced with this exact battle before.

I'm glad to say, Larry and I rode out that storm and the Lord helped me get control over it. Once I was over that, I started some real thinking about my relationship with my husband. Just recently I became aware of all those walls I had built around myself for protection. I realized I had never really loved anyone in the true sense of the word and it was time I started to learn. I'm starting to reach out a little at a time. Larry and I are beginning to talk, and he's saying more as I become less defensive.

I have been able to admit that believing and accepting his love is difficult, that giving myself to him has been a half-done job, that rejection scares me. I think we have both faced the fact that because of many things in each of our lives we have built barriers, and we have both felt persecuted and unloved and dissatisfied. We agree we have a lot of work to do. But if God has helped me through everything else, He can certainly teach me how to love genuinely and to allow give and take in my marriage. It is beginning to happen, and I have never felt better about our marriage than I do now.

My parents feel I've changed, that I'm really not the same person, and they are thrilled with the changes. After all the years of fighting about my weight, my mother and I can now wear each other's clothes. My father is bursting his buttons, just as if I were being born all over again. I saw him a couple of months ago for the first time in a year. To him the change was quite dramatic.

The people I work with, of course, have witnessed these changes on a day-to-day basis. I don't think they even realize how much I've gone through right under their noses. They will admit I'm not the same person who came to work there four years ago. Over and over again, they have seen me rush into the office to announce that my new dress is one size smaller. They have seen me live through hungry days, easy days, happy days, and some of those days when I wondered if it was worth it. Some of them miss the old me now and then. They miss some of the three-ring circuses I used to put on, and they feel I have become a little too quiet. But basically they approve of what they see. But whether they approve or not is not the important thing. I want to tell you what I think of myself.

I like me. I like what's happening to me. See, the most important thing is not the weight loss, but what is happening as a result of it. By getting rid of those pounds and that image of myself as a failure—as an ugly, unlovable person—I have gotten out from under the one thing that shaped my thinking on everything.

I want you to meet the new Karen Wise, as seen by Karen Wise. I hope you feel you have never met her before, although she bears some resemblance to the girl in all the other chapters.

She is not a bad person. She is a human being

filled with dreams and desires and emotions and abilities. She makes mistakes and stumbles occasionally, but she is a child of God and is learning more each day to depend on Him for wisdom, guidance, warmth, and new attitudes. She has a lot of worth. God created her in a very special way, as He creates everyone, to fill a very special place in His world. She is a performer at heart and loves to be in front of people. She loves music and drama and writing and directing and feels good about having these interests. She is attractive and is beginning to really think thin instead of fat.

She is much more relaxed because she doesn't have to prove anything to the people around her. She is nicer to be around because she isn't always trying to compensate, and she is so much quieter and far less overbearing. Her whole spirit seems to be different. There is a mellowness and a gentleness that was never there before. She is fun. She laughs and joins in and comes out with funny lines, but she doesn't have to be the one telling the jokes.

She is finding it easier to talk to people and to make friends, and the attitude of other people toward her is also different. She is far more secure than she used to be and much less defensive. She is actually getting to the place where she can accept criticism without feeling that she is being attacked personally. She is working at becoming a better wife and mother because she believes she is loved and that she has the ability to love in return. Getting one hundred percent approval from Christian society is not her goal. God's approval seems far more important. She is not a misfit. Rather, she is an individual who is finally, with God's help, fitting herself together.

I hope you like her. I do.

When people ask me what is the best thing about losing weight, most of them expect me to say buying clothes or being able to fit into a chair. These things are terrific, but there is one thing that outshines everything else—the ability to be comfortable around other people.

I still catch myself outside a room with my hand on the doorknob, dreading going in where there is a group of people I don't know. I stand there and secretly hope the vacant chair will be nearest the door so I won't have to walk in front of people. And then I have to say to myself, "For goodness' sake, Karen, open the door and walk in. You don't have to be embarrassed to walk across the room. You look good now. Remember?" And to walk into that room, find my chair, sit down, cross my legs, and feel comfortable and accepted for what I am is the greatest privilege in my new world.

Losing weight has only been a beginning. Because I feel better about myself, a lot of other healing is taking place as a result. I am finding it much easier to trust—to trust God and to trust other people as well. A great deal of my cynicism is beginning to disappear. I am not as quick to point my finger or criticize other people. I am no longer depending on the status of other people to justify or intimidate mine. I have also learned that there is a big difference between human bravery and trust in God. I have lived through some real crises as a Christian, and I have been brave and shown others I am brave; but I hassled and fought and pushed to get through them. How much easier and beneficial it is to trust God to help you work out the answer, and you don't damage so many others in the process.

I am no longer angry or bitter. What a difference this has made in my disposition and total personality. I will always be a person with strong opinions and definite ideas, but I no longer strike out just because I am mad or feel cheated or boxed in. The most significant change, however, is that I now enjoy being a Christian. When I became a Christian I knew God accepted me and loved me the way I was, but I also knew He would be much more pleased if we licked my weight problem. I have always carried a load of guilt around—guilt about my past and my weight and my failure to do something about it. But now my relationship with the Lord is changing because that heavy load of guilt is gone. My past is only brought up if it can help someone else. It is not brought up every day to haunt me. What is done is done. I can't undo it. Just as God has given total forgiveness, He also has given me—finally—the ability to forgive myself. That was the hardest lesson to learn. I didn't have to keep punishing myself. It was over.

My feelings about the Christian world and about being a Christian have also changed. I was reading in Galatians one morning and all of a sudden I realized I have always felt to one degree or another a slave to Christianity instead of a free individual in Christ. Even after I was born again, I spent a lot of time trying to meet all the "Christian" standards, and I continued to come up short. I wasn't in trouble anymore and I was existing well in Christian society. But I wasn't really enjoying the fact that I had the freedom to become what God intended me to become. I didn't have to live under the pressure of feeling that I had to be exactly like the Christian next to me, or across the aisle, or in the second pew in order to be genuinely spiritual.

With this realization, I quit working so hard at trying to fit and accepted myself as God made me. Immediately, I became more comfortable, and I found I had a lot more in common with most Christians than what I had thought. When I differed with other Christians, I could accept the difference, remain secure, and not have it damage my view of them or everyone else.

The funny thing is, I still don't really fit into every place and with everybody in the Christian world. But I have found I don't want to be a "complete fitter" anyway. I would rather fit snugly into that special niche God has for me, reaching those people I can reach and having the ministry God has planned for me.

So often we forget that God created each one of us individually. He didn't mass produce anybody. And He deals with us each differently. He gives each of us the opportunity to fulfill a unique spot in His plan.

It is that opportunity I am taking today— working at my marriage, improving the relationship with my children, and reaching out and learning to give and take love and friendship and understanding. And I'm growing a lot. Not *around,* but *up* this time. That's it really. With God's help I am finally growing up.

All through my life I have prayed for help of one kind or another. I have prayed in anger, and I have told God to get off my back. My prayer is quite different today.

"Thank You for Your patience and Your love for me.

"Thank You for giving me the opportunity and the strength I needed to acquire courage, self-discipline, and endurance.

"Thank You for liking me and for showing me how to like myself. And thank You most of all for Your total forgiveness and my bright future as Your child.

"Keep Your hand on me. Keep me thin by keeping my priorities in order.

"Thank You for my husband, my children, my parents, my sister, and for all those in the body of Christ who loved me and prayed for me along the way. Amen."

CHAPTER 12

A WORD FROM THE WISE

I hope you are not reading this chapter first, because you need to know what I've lived through before you read my suggestions. I believe my past experiences give credibility to what I have to say.

I would like to pass on some things that might help you if you are overweight or if you are the parent of a fat child. I also have a few hints for Christian parents who have children who are giving you a "run for your money," as they say.

First, if you are overweight, here are a few things that I feel will be most helpful:

1. Quit blaming everybody else for your problem. It's yours . . . totally yours. You are the one who ate the food. You have to take off the weight.

2. Sit down and write out how being overweight affects your life-style, your appearance, your family, your friends, and your attitude about yourself. This will help you to see how severe the problem is.

3.   Don't wait for the right time to diet. If you are looking for that special day when there will be no upsets, problems, pressures, or emotional conflicts, it will probably never come. God is strong enough to help you do it today.

4.   Go on a diet just for you. If you go on a diet for anybody else, you will depend too heavily on their encouragement. If you don't get the encouragement, you'll quit. Only when you do it for you will it work.

5.   Ask for God's help. Ask Him to change the priority in your life from food to what He wants you to be. Tell Him you can't do it by yourself, that He will have to give you some qualities you don't have. But don't quit praying there. Pray often. Pray when you are in any situation where your hands start to move for more butter or your mouth begins to water for a chocolate milkshake. Pray hardest when you are standing in front of the refrigerator with the door open. And don't forget to thank Him when you close it—contents untouched. Oh, and one more thing about praying. God can't lose the weight for you, either. When you've prayed for help, remember that it takes the combination of God's qualities and your action. Praying won't take the pounds off unless you lock

yourself in the prayer closet without any food for a long time.

6. Keep busy. Get out of the house. This is particularly important at first. If someone is an alcoholic and is trying to quit, you don't drive him down to the corner bar at 8:00 in the morning and tell him to sit there and not drink until you pick him up at 5:00. If you have a bad food problem, don't park yourself by the refrigerator all day. Find a job; take the kids to the park, do volunteer work; go for a walk. But keep busy and keep moving.

7. Find a diet that works for you and that you can live with. The same diet doesn't work for everybody. Just as our life-styles differ, so does the diet program we can each realistically stick with. And don't play around with it. Don't go on it for a few days and off it for a few days. You will never get over the hump that way. Your cravings will never lessen, and your body will never get to the place where it adapts, if you don't stick to it everyday.

8. Don't play games with yourself. Don't waste the time rationalizing that one dessert or a homemade biscuit won't hurt you. It works against the weight loss and worse than that, it revives your cravings

for those things. Once you cheat, you will find it harder to turn those things down the next time.

9. Watch out for the people who try to ruin your diet. Don't let them talk you into eating. They will try, and they will come up with good reasons to give in. Don't ever think they are doing you a favor.

10. Try to eat your main meal at noon and eat light for supper. You may have to work at that a little, and you may even have to learn to watch other people eat while you have nothing, but it can be done and you will lose a lot quicker that way. One word of warning: Don't make those around you feel uncomfortable. Pretend it doesn't bother you and pretty soon, it won't.

11. If you fall on your face and go on a binge, start again the next day. Don't tell yourself you're a failure. If the binges come every other day, however, you might as well admit that you aren't on a diet.

12. Talk to yourself. Instead of telling yourself you will never make it, start saying you *are* going to make it. Replace those awful thoughts about yourself with some verbal affirmations. That will help you mentally as well as physically.

13.   Every time you change sizes, buy at least one thing that fits. This will do wonders for you, and it will also help other people notice your progress. And when others begin to notice, you will be encouraged.

14.   Don't make food your reward for dieting, and don't let other people reward you that way. Food is not a reward—it is your enemy. I hear many people say that when they lose so much weight, they are going to treat themselves to a hot fudge sundae; or they say their husband told them that if they lose ten pounds, he will take them out for an expensive steak dinner. Food is still too important to you, if you use it as a reward.

You have probably heard most of these things before. I don't have any new information or tricks up my sleeve. I knew all of these things, too, years before I put them into practice. My saying them won't make any difference to you either if you are not really ready to tackle the problem. But when you are ready, keep these things in mind.

Let me say one important thing. You do not have to be 200 pounds overweight to have a severe problem. I meet people regularly who are only twenty to thirty pounds overweight, but are just as bothered by it as I was by my 225 pounds of excess weight. They talk about it every day. They hate the way they look; they don't have anything to wear;

their husbands or wives are nagging them to take it off. Every day they say they are going to go on a diet. The problem is constantly on their minds. If this is the case with you, you have a problem. Even though it's not as big as mine was, it is definitely affecting your whole life.

Let me say one more thing. The Christian world is almost the hardest place to exist when you are on a diet. We are extremely food oriented. Wherever there is a group of Christians, there is usually a chocolate cake or a ham sandwich. Eating is our only sanctioned vice. I am sure you realize that the *true* definition of fellowship is eating with one another. Between church potlucks, Sunday school class dinners, Valentine banquets, annual picnics, receptions, after-every-meeting-get-togethers, Bible studies with refreshments, men's breakfasts and ladies' teas—the weak, overeating Christian doesn't stand a ghost of a chance. We don't know how to do anything else. We even entice people to go visiting by telling them that afterwards we will return to the church for hot chocolate and dough-nuts in the winter and cookies and lemonade in the summer. Overweight Christians love to stand around and talk about people who smoke, drink, and go to night clubs, while they are eating their second piece of pie.

If you are living in that world, be ready for it and realize that you just can't let it get to you.

I do understand what it is like to have a weight problem and not to be able to do anything about it. I haven't forgotten the struggle and the pain. I am reminded each time I look in the mirror of what I have done to my body. But I am living proof that God can make a difference, that He can help you get control over your eating habits. I encourage you to give Him the opportunity to do for you what He has done for me.

If you are battling a slight weight problem, I hope you have decided after reading this book to never let happen to you what happened to me. Take off the thirty pounds before it becomes forty or fifty or sixty. Believe me, you don't want to live like that.

Now, if you are the parent of a fat child, I hope you have already benefited from this book. Let me list the things I feel you need to know and remember.

1. Even though you want to, you cannot demand or make your child lose weight. Face that, and you will be over a big hurdle.

2. Keep your mouth shut. Try hard not to nag about the problem. Put a piece of tape over your mouth if you have to, but don't stay on his back. Nagging only makes him mad. It will ruin any chance you have to really communicate with your child, even on other subjects.

3. Accept the child for what he is. Don't make him think you love him any less because he is fat. He needs you to love him just the way he is. But remember,

there is a difference between love and
indulgence.

4. Build his self-esteem. Major on his posi-
tive points. If he thinks he's worthwhile,
he will someday think enough of himself
to help himself.

5. Do everything you can to help your child
look as good as he can, even though he is
fat. Some parents get so irritated by the
weight and so frustrated in trying to find
clothes, they take the attitude that the
child is going to look bad anyway, so why
work at trying to help what can't be
helped. Try to choose the right clothes
and encourage good grooming. Again, this
makes for a better self-image.

6. Remember that the fat person is very
much aware of his problem and of his in-
adequacies. You don't have to list them for
him.

7. When the child is upset because he has
been treated cruelly or has been left out or
rejected because of his weight, help him
to realize that is his responsibility. He ate
the food; he has to cope with the con-
sequences. And don't offer him a piece of
cake and a glass of milk to make him feel
better.

8. If you have never had a weight problem yourself, don't keep telling the child you understand, because you don't—and they know it. You will get further if you tell them you don't understand, but you love them and are willing to help them in any way you can. Don't be an authority on weight loss if you have never been on a diet.

9. Let the child suggest a diet; don't put him on one against his will. This will only teach him to sneak food. In the long run, he will eat more.

10. Do not make him feel guilty for every bite of food he eats at home. If you do, he will arrange ways of staying out of your sight while he eats. No one ever hides to eat fruits or vegetables. Therefore, the more the child hides and sneaks, be assured the more junk food he is eating.

11. When he does go on a diet, help him, encourage him, but don't give him the third degree.

12. When the child quits dieting, don't make him think he is a failure as a total person because he couldn't stick with it. Enough endorsed and underlined failures will convince him not to try anymore.

13.   Be sure you notice every little bit of progress when he diets successfully. Reinforce his abilities and strengths, and tell him you can tell he is losing. Buy him new clothes when he changes even one size, and tell him you are proud of him. CAUTION: Don't overdo it. If you do, he will conclude you really don't like him if he's fat; and if he fails and gains the weight back, he will remember that.

There are four things I would like to say to parents of small children who might have the tendency to put on weight. These four things may work as preventive medicine to a certain degree.

1.   *Do not make your child clean his plate if he is full.* Give him a good balanced meal and don't give him huge servings. When he is full let him quit with the understanding that he doesn't come back for more in an hour or that he doesn't quit just to save room for cake. Don't lay that stuff about the starving Orientals on him. Simply let him leave the excess food. Why make them stretch their stomachs?

2.   *Don't serve dessert with every meal.* Pretty soon, no meal is complete without it. It's surprising how one can live without dessert. And snacks don't have to be candy or potato chips. A snack can consist

of raisins, an apple, a cracker, or frozen yogurt just as well.

3. *Don't use food as a reward* for being good or making good grades or not kicking the babysitter. There are other options, you know. This reward stuff is a bad pattern to set.

4. (I should star this one. It is very important). *Don't create the habit of eating before bed.* A lot of children think of this as a part of their regular routine, and a lot of adults are struggling through those before-bedtime hours trying to break the habit their parents started years before. Have supper and leave it at that.

I have two children, and many times I wonder how I will handle it if one of them has a severe weight problem. I don't know all the answers. However I have put these things into practice in my own home. I don't know if these hints will help in your particular situation, but I share them knowing there is a possibility they will help someone. (If they don't, my mother might be available for consultation!)

This next list of suggestions is to Christian parents living with their families in a Christian world.

1. I know you have heard this before: Replace the negative with positives. Instead

of having an eighteen-year-old who is able to recite the list of things he can't do, why not see that he is able to recite a list of all the benefits he has in knowing Jesus Christ as Savior.

2.   Don't make everything so important that when the genuinely important things come along, he doesn't hear you. What do you want him to remember, the ten reasons why he didn't go to the senior prom or the practical ways that Christ becomes a reality in his everyday life?

3.   Don't set yourself up as a spiritual giant. When your weaknesses show, they will stick out like a sore thumb. Admit you're still growing, that you make mistakes, that God is still working on you. Be real—not programmed.

4.   Don't get so busy with church that it takes the place of the time you should be spending with your family.

5.   Don't assume that taking a child to church regularly means you are building a good spiritual foundation. You might be very surprised too late.

6.   Whatever personality and talents God has given your child, let him know God didn't make a mistake. Admittedly, the rough

edges need to be smoothed out, but don't ever think the whole package was wrong. And don't squelch the talent—find an outlet for it. God has a purpose for that talent.

7. Don't raise the child in such a protected church environment that he has trouble relating what he has learned in the "real" world. You want him to be an effective Christian in the world. You do not want him to run from it and hide, or run to it to escape.

8. Do not pressure your children into making a lot of public spiritual decisions. Let God handle conviction. The motive for a pressured decision is less than terrific, and usually not lasting.

9. Try to understand the reason for outward behavior. Don't just attack what you see happening. Try to find what's going on inside.

10. Don't ever make a child feel that the way to really please you is by going into full-time Christian service. The person who is a missionary or a preacher or a youth director because he feels that's the only way to effectively serve God shouldn't be there. A Christian businessman, a Christian school teacher, a Christian lawyer, or a Christian musician can have a marvelous

ministry reaching people no preacher could ever reach. A full-time ministry position is wonderful, but only if that is what God really wants you to do.

11. We can't escape it, parents, you and I. The most important thing is to live what you say you believe. Everything else amounts to zero without this.

You don't have to be perfect, but don't tell your children you are, either.

You can make mistakes, but show them God has helped you learn from them.

Let your children watch you grow in the Lord. Don't let them watch you stagnate. Show them you enjoy being a Christian and that it's a marvelous way to live. Don't let it appear dull, uninteresting, and boxed in. Make it the kind of life that they will be able to look at and say, "That's what I want."

Let the reality of Christ show in your marriage and in your love and support of your children. Let it show in your personality and your business dealings and in your friendships.

You are the best evidence of what you want your children to believe or not believe in.

I agree that's scary! But it's also true.

I pray that I, as a parent, will continually point my children to Jesus Christ—through my life, my progress, and my acceptance and love for them.

Well, that's my story, my advice, my testimony of what God has done with a fat preacher's kid.

It hasn't been a pretty story, but maybe you're not in a pretty place, and just perhaps you saw yourself on a page or two. If so, remember this: I don't have the corner on God's miracles. I'm sure He can perform one in you if you are willing to let Him work in your life.

"We made it this time, didn't we, Lord?"